A Dynamic Materia Medica of the Noble Gases

KRYPTON

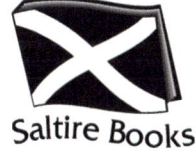

Saltire Books *Saltire Books Limited, Glasgow, Scotland*

A Dynamic Materia Medica of the Noble Gases

KRYPTON

Jeremy Sherr

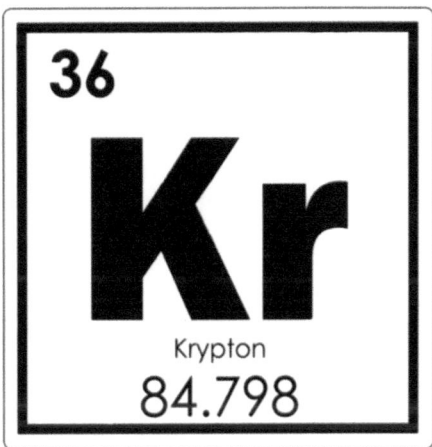

Saltire Books   *Saltire Books Limited, Glasgow, Scotland*

Published by Saltire Books Ltd

18–20 Main Street, Busby, Glasgow G76 8DU, Scotland
books@saltirebooks.com   www.saltirebooks.com

Cover, Design, Layout and Text © Saltire Books Ltd 2024
Poems copyright J Sherr unless otherwise attributed

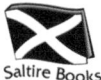 is a registered trademark

First published in 2024

Typeset by Type Study, Scarborough, UK in 9.25pt on 13.5pt Stone Serif
Printed and bound in the UK by TJ Books Ltd, Padstow, Cornwall

ISBN 978-1-908127-17-4

For Saltire
Project Development: Lee Kayne
Editorial: Steven Kayne
Designer: Phil Barker
Indexee: Laurence Errington
Illustrator: Matt Canning

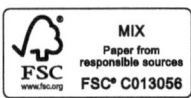

CONTENTS

Dedicated to my son Ike Daniel Sherr, who has a beautiful heart and knows almost everything

Teach me Lord, a blessing and a prayer
The mystery of a wilting leaf, of radiant ripening fruit
And freedom thus: to see, to sense, inhale
To know, to yearn and fail
Instruct my lips a blessing, song of praise
As you renew each evening and each day
And so my times shall never be the same
Nor habit spoil my living breathing day

What Man has written, Leah Goldberg[1]

I had the good fortune of having Edward Whitmont, the well-known homoeopath and Jungian psychoanalyst, as a friend. Once, over sushi in our favourite New York restaurant, I asked him my million-dollar question: 'What is the solution to the problem of time?' His first answer was: 'There is no answer; there was no answer; and there will be no answer'. Then, after some reflection, he said: "There is one thing. Prioritise."

If I had not listened to his advice, you would not be reading this book.

JS

*There was a joke when I woke Four cons = it was cryptic. Con cave was the cave a con? A "C" is a quarter of an "8". Dismember the * and you get four C's.*

Krypton proving[2]

What is God? He is length, width, height and depth.

St. Bernard of Clairvaux[3]

(And time – JS)

Apple fall, Newton call
Eins-time moving on,
We're diving through the mirror now
And heading for Krypton

Keppler counting, Rabbi blessing
Moon and sun revolve
Six and thirty puzzles here
That you cannot re-solve

Superman or batman?
Joker or a riddle?
The period we visit next
Is lying in the middle.

Chambers pumping, heart is beating
One, two, three and four
Dali Lama, hieroglyphics,
Who could ask for more?

ACKNOWLEDGMENTS

A proving is a product of many people acting As If One Person, and so is this book. My thanks and gratitude go to the following friends and colleagues, without whom this book would not and could not manifest.

To the lovely students of Dynamis London 1996, who formed a happy group.

To Gabriella Reiberer, Loretta August, Denise, Marlise, for editing the proving.

Thanks to Silvie Gowen for her extraordinary provings and her dedication in recording them. Once again Silvie has intercepted the subtle codes of universal consciousness in a most remarkable way.

To John Morgan from Helios pharmacy for preparing the remedy and for supporting the noble art of proving.

To Yocheved Abram, Rose Nightingale, Tina Quirk, Wenda O'Reilly and Rebecca Stirrup for proof reading, editing and advice.

Special thanks to Tina for excellent work in referencing this book.

Thanks to Dr. Chris Kurz for 4th dimensional advice.

To Francis Treuherz for Lewis Carroll. To Andreas Bjørndal for review.

To Joanne Greenland, Rebecca Stirrup and Sharon Wells, for supporting me in writing this book.

To Joel Jaffe, my trusted video editor who produces the most wonderful moving images. May he rest in peace.

To Jurek Dabrowski for Krypton substance report.

To all those who sent cases: Camilla Sherr, Doug Brown, Denise Straiges.

To my spiritual mentor Yaakov Melamed Cohen.

To my publishers Steven and Lee Kayne of Saltire Books Limited, Glasgow.

To all my good friends, colleagues, and students who have supported me through the years. You are all part of my journey, and I of yours. Each one of you has been so good to me, for me, for homoeopathy. I thank you with all my heart.

To my wife Camilla for being my muse.

ABOUT THE AUTHOR

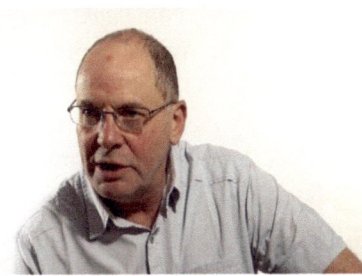 **Jeremy Sherr** has practised and taught homoeopathy internationally since 1980. He is founder of 'The Dynamis School for Advanced Homoeopathic Studies', the longest running postgraduate course in the world.

He has conducted 45 classical homoeopathic provings and is the author of *The Dynamics and Methodology of Homoeopathic Provings, Dynamic Materia Medica – Syphilis, Dynamic Provings Volumes I and II, The Repertory of Mental Qualities, and The Dynamic Materia Medica of the Noble Gases – Helium, Neon, and Argon*, and the forthcoming *Adaptive Translation of the Organon*, and the *Dynamic Treatment of Epidemics*. He has published numerous articles on homoeopathy and has conducted several research programmes. In addition to his homoeopathy credentials, Jeremy holds a degree in traditional Chinese medicine and has honorary professorships in several international universities.

Since 2008 Jeremy and his wife Camilla have been living in Tanzania where they have organised rural clinics and are working in local hospitals. They have treated tens of thousands of AIDS and other patients with classical homoeopathy, set up educational and food programs, and established a day care centre for children with AIDS.

In December 2022, Jeremy published his first middle-grade fiction title, *The Noble Adventures of Beryl and Carol* for which he was awarded the Pencraft Best Book Award 2024, the Children's book international best adventure and best bedtime story 2024.

ILLUSTRATION CREDITS

Figure 2.1 Krypton in the periodic table. *J Sherr Saltire Books.*

Figure 2.2 Krypton atomic structure. *Wikipedia.* Available online at: http://tinyurl.com/2d2wwuwx (accessed July 18, 2023).

Figure 6.1 Superman in action *Superman comic Issue number 1*. Chicago: Consolidated Book Publishers. Summer, 1939. Available online at: http://tinyurl.com/2tzfdku6 (accessed March 12, 2024).

Figure 7.1 Leopard clothing: Ksenia Chernaya. *Pexels Photos.* Available online at: http://tinyurl.com/yc8n6bcy (accessed March 12, 2024).

Figure 8.1 Karnak Temple. *Shutterstock.* Available online at: http://tinyurl.com/yr5mbuzr (accessed March 12, 2024).

Figure 8.2 Osiris. Statues. *Shutterstock.* Available online at: http://tinyurl.com/53v6hj9y (accessed March 12, 2024).

Figure 8.3 Eye of Horus In: ReFaey K, Quinones GC, Tripathy S. The Eye of Horus: The Connection between Art, Medicine and Mythology in Ancient Egypt. *Cureus* 2019; 11(5). Available online at: http://tinyurl.com/4pxydk2x (accessed March 12, 2024).

Figure 8.4 Day four of Creation. *Produced by Saltire Books.*

Figure 8.5 Curved space-time creating gravity. *Shutterstock.* Available online at: http://tinyurl.com/3yswkesz and http://tinyurl.com/ya66rz3a (accessed March 18, 2024).

Figure 9.1 The Thinker. (Rodin). *Image. static flickr.* Available online at: http://tinyurl.com/2mhjxbuw (accessed March 13, 2024).

Figure 9.2 Harmony separating into line and circle. *J Sherr.*

Figure 10.1 Vertical alignment of the noble elements. *J Sherr.*

Figure 10.2 Giacometti woman. *Image. static flickr.* Available online at: http://tinyurl.com/yj3577a8 (accessed March 13, 2024).

Figure 10.3 Angles of the periodic table. *J Sherr.*

Figure 10.4 Krypton Kross. *J Sherr.*

Figure 10.5 The celestial equator. *Shutterstock.* Available online at: http://tinyurl.com/msencwec (accessed March 21, 2024).

Figure 10.6 Longitudes and Latitudes. Available online at: http://tinyurl. com/3bbme3mu and http://tinyurl.com/mrkfpptc (accessed July 18, 2023). *Redrawn by Saltire Books.*

Figure 10.7 Mercator projection. *Fineart. America.* Available online at: http://tinyurl.com/4zhmwezn (accessed March 13, 2024).

Figure 10.8 Surface area of a sphere: Line curving. *Study.com.* Available online at: http://tinyurl.com/mpfn54xc (accessed July 18, 2023).

Figure 10.9 Sphere moving into fourth dimension time. *J Sherr Saltire Books.*

Figure 10.10 Superman curving time. *World of Krypton* Edition 1. July, 1979. Chicago: Grand Comics Database. Available online at: http://tinyurl. com/4jeeep7v (accessed March 13, 2024).

Figure 10.11 Tree of life pathways. *J Sherr Saltire Books.*

Figure 11.1 Time as a continuum. Available online at: http://tinyurl.com/ 2v4vfrk7 (accessed July 18, 2023). *Redrawn by Saltire Books.*

Figure 11.2 4D life. *Pixobay.* Available online at: http://tinyurl.com/ 3kj24m6u (accessed July 18, 2023). *Redrawn by Saltire Books.*

Figure 11.3 Four dimensions. *Produced by Saltire Books.*

Figure 11.4 Each dimension creates the next one. Available online at: http://tinyurl.com/yckf9wm2 (accessed July 18, 2023). *Redrawn by Saltire Books.*

Figure 11.5 Time perpendicular to space. Available online at: http:// tinyurl.com/yckf9wm2 (accessed July 18, 2023). *Redrawn by Saltire Books.*

Figure 11.6 Allagappan S. The Timeless Journey of the Möbius Strip. *Scientific American* January 14, 2021. Available online at: http://tinyurl. com/3xwk47w8 (accessed July 18, 2023). *Produced by Saltire Books.*

Figure 11.7 Spacetime curving. *Shutterstock.* Available online at: http:// tinyurl.com/4p3h87ye (accessed March 13, 2024).

Figure 11.8 Development of spacetime structure. *J Sherr Saltire Books.*

Figure 12.1 Krypton from Wordle cloud generator. Available online at: http://tinyurl.com/3bhmevxu (accessed July 18, 2023).

Figure 14.1 Kryptonian alphabet 42 *Omniglot online encyclopaedia.* Available online at: http://tinyurl.com/yzp4779k (accessed July 18, 2023).

Figure 14.2 DNA synthesising. *J Sherr Saltire Books.*

Figure 14.3 DNA Splitting and replication. Gustafsso M. Hörnquist M. Coherent waves in DNA within the Peyrard-Bishop model. *Research Gate,* October 2011. Available online at: http://tinyurl.com/bdwjvdvh (accessed March 13, 2024).

Figure 14.4 mRNA forming mirror images with tRNA. Greenwood S Protein Synthesis-Translation.png: mRNA. *Wikimedia Commons.* Available online at: http://tinyurl.com/w6zmeshb (accessed July 18, 2023).

18.11E Pickpik. Available online at: http://tinyurl.com/wswfhepk (accessed March 14, 2024).

18.11F Images-wixmp. Available online at: http://tinyurl.com/3pwe8wyx (accessed March 14, 2024).

Figure 18.12 Mann GN. *Yeat's Vision.* Available online at: http://www.yeatsvision.com/Geometry.html (accessed July 18, 2023).

Figure 18.13 Vortex 13. *Diagrams by Walter Russell,* courtesy of the University of Science & Philosophy, http://www.philosophy.org/#/ (accessed March 15, 2024).

Figure 18.14 Electric coil. *Diagram by Walter Russell, idem.*

Figure 18.15 Gyroscope. *Diagram by Walter Russell, idem.*

Figure 18.16 Double gyre. *Diagram by Walter Russell, idem.*

Figure 18.17 Double coils. *Diagram by Walter Russell W, idem.*

Figure 18.18 Principal Symbol. Yeats WB. *A Vision. Expectations and Contexts.* Liverpool: Liverpool University Press 2012. Available online at: http://tinyurl.com/3rt9z5wv (accessed March 15, 2024).

PREFACE

What man has written, man may read,
But God fills every root and seed,
With cryptic words,
To strangely set,
For mortals to decipher yet.

Charles Dalman[4]

This book has several aims. Other than teaching the remedy Krypton, it carries on the journey of the noble gases, which in turn illuminates the entire periodic table. Furthermore, this is a practical manual of how to turn a proving into Materia Medica, to learn how to weave the web of meaning and perceive the connection on every possible level. Yes, it is hard work. But learn how to do it once, and it will help all your remedy and case analyses and syntheses, the route to mastery.

Krypton is a remedy for our times. It is one of the most fascinating remedies that I have ever proved, providing many clues to the secrets of the universe, space and time, mind, language, and our inner nature, if only we can decipher the code. It is also one of the most intellectually demanding. So, get the wheels of your brain revolving, as we set out on the cryptic journey of Krypton.

After each proving at the Dynamis School we hold a provers' meeting at which the provers and supervisors recount their experiences. At the end of this process, and before revealing the substance, I ask the class to guess the remedy, a riddle for the homoeopathic mind. The prize for those who find the correct answer is a meal in the restaurant of their choice. I offer this prize with some confidence, as it is extremely rare that anyone comes up with the right remedy, or even the kingdom to which it belongs. This highlights the weakness of the doctrine of signatures and kingdoms. The remedy picture produced by a proving does not, and should not, directly resemble the external nature of the substance proved; for we are dealing with the obscure world of metaphor and analogy, the encrypted world of inner structure and simple substance. A proving is conducted to elicit the unexpected, not the expected.

Of all the remedies I have proved it would have to be Krypton which trashed my neat logical theory, resulting in me buying five smug provers expensive meals in a top Scottish restaurant (involving wild salmon and much good whiskey). To be fair four of these solved the riddle by means of intellectual deduction rather than the experience. They knew I was on the noble gas journey, and which remedies I had already proved, so it was a matter of putting two and two together. The fifth however, declared it was Superman's blood, a purely intuitive conjecture which took me by surprise. Until today I do not know how she got this idea, but I guess there is always a fifth intuitive to four's logic.

The proving of Krypton was conducted at Dynamis London in 1996, in parallel to the proving of Argon in Dynamis Ireland. It was a jolly group of provers, yet the experience was far from that of the joyful Argon, and while some provers scaled the lofty peaks of spiritual experience, where past and present meet in the now, others recycled time's weary treadmill. My own proving of Krypton was a bleak and devastating experience, in which my wife and I felt disconnected from ourselves, from each other, from love and from God. It was a desperate sensation of hopelessly and helplessly sliding down the slippery slopes of chronic disease, with the certain knowledge that there could be no return to our previous loving and blissful state.

There is an old joke: When someone asks 'do you have a match?', you reply 'not since Superman'. I must admit to not being an intellectual match for Krypton's many secrets. It is not an easy remedy. Rather, it is a complex, complicated enigma which requires cerebral courage and mental labour to fully fathom. Krypton throws a 'curved ball' at one's brain and it can mess with your computer. To fully understand its riddles, I would need to be a scholar of many disciplines of which I have but a cursory knowledge: Maths, Geometry, Navigation, Tibetan Buddhism, Egyptology, and Encryption. I have tried to scratch the surface where I could, and I leave further investigations to those more knowledgeable than myself.

Jeremy Sherr
Tanzania
February 1st 2024

References

1   Goldberg, L. Teach Me. Rachel and Leah (translated from Hebrew by Jeremy Sherr). p11. Available online at: http://tinyurl.com/bdeav3z4 (accessed February 20, 2024).
2   The proving of Krypton was conducted at Dynamis London in 1996.
3   Saint Bernard of Clairvaux. In: *Consideration*. Aeterna Press 2015. Quote available online at: http://tinyurl.com/5xb8byjx (accessed July 18, 2023).
4   Dalmon CW. Research Database of Authors. Available online at: http://tinyurl.com/ye22f9na (accessed February 20, 2024).

1

INTRODUCTION

The potencies of perception

In this book, as in the rest of this series covering the noble gases, I equate the chapter name with levels of perception corresponding to the scale of potencies.

This is an analogy and has absolutely nothing to do with potencies proved or to the potencies to be used in clinical cases.

The potency should be selected according to the totality of the case regardless of in which chapter the symptom lies.

Starting with a very basic understanding of the chemical element and its preparation on the mother tincture level, the chapters ascend the potencies of perception through affinity, keynote and emotional essence, rising to the higher potencies of geometrical structure, physical dimensions and collective concepts.

Here is a summary of levels of potency equated with levels of perception, ranging from the gross to the subtle:

- The mother tincture represents homoeopathic preparation, the realm of atoms and molecules.
- The 12C level represents physical affinities, the realm of organs.
- The 30C represents general themes, the realm of the organism.
- The 200C represents a simple emotional 'essence'.
- The 1M is a more detailed description of the mental emotional symptom configuration in a search of a unified understanding.
- The 10M describes the more subtle spiritual aspects of the proving, including a very astute meditation proving.
- The 50M represents subtle sensations and functions, including the numerological and geometrical structure of the remedy, and its relation to the physical dimensions.
- The CM explores the world of analogy and metaphor.
- The MM and beyond are an investigation into the esoteric roots of the remedy and the universal blueprint that lies beyond.

According to my 'grammatical' method of analysis described in my book, *Syphilis*,[1] the 12C and 30C chapters correspond to nouns; the 200C and 1M represent adjectives and adverbs; and the 50M and above stands for verbs, movement in time and space. The potencies beyond touch the language of philosophy and poetry. Matching the remedy to the patient on the higher potencies of similarity will lead to deeper results. However, for optimum similarity, all levels should fit.

I do not intend these correspondences to be precise, rather a general idea. Creating yet another system to which homoeopaths should strictly adhere can only lead to rigid thinking and prescribing.

I have included some cases after the 50M chapter because most Krypton cases can be solved from knowledge gained from previous chapters. The higher levels of the CM chapter and above relate to broader concepts than the individual remedy.

Only selected quotes from the provings have found their way into each section; many symptoms only appear in the unabridged proving document. It is important to read the proving as a whole to gain a thorough understanding of the remedy. The full proving may be found at www.dynamis.edu.

When capitalised, *Krypton* refers to homoeopathic remedies, while *krypton* with a lower-case *k* refer to the chemical element. All original symptoms from the Krypton proving are given as follows: Krypton symptom. Some proving symptoms have been abbreviated or grammar has been corrected without changing the essential content. The complete and original text can be found in the proving text itself. Keywords and phrases that I consider important are occasionally marked **in bold** within the proving.

Note: More than in most other remedies, Krypton symptoms may be understood at different levels, hence there will be repetition of some symptoms as we ascend the potencies of perception.

Reference

1   Sherr J. *Syphilis* (2nd edn, reprint). Glasgow: Saltire Books, 2021.

2

KRYPTON: THE ELEMENT

The symbol for Krypton is Kr, with the atomic number 36, and atomic weight 83.80. Krypton belongs to group 0 of the periodic table (see Figure 2.1). The name Krypton comes from the Greek word *kryptos*, which means hidden. It is one of six known noble gases: helium (He), neon (Ne), argon (Ar), krypton (Kr), xenon (Xe) and radon (Rn), and a possible seventh – the elusive element 118, which I have termed luciferium, (but which the International Union of Pure and Applied Chemistry has named 'oganesson' The name honours the Russian nuclear physicist Yuri Oganessian, who played a leading role in the discovery of the heaviest elements in the periodic table.[1]

Composition

The *noble gases* exist under normal conditions as colourless, odourless, tasteless non-flammable gases. The gases were thought to be rare, however,

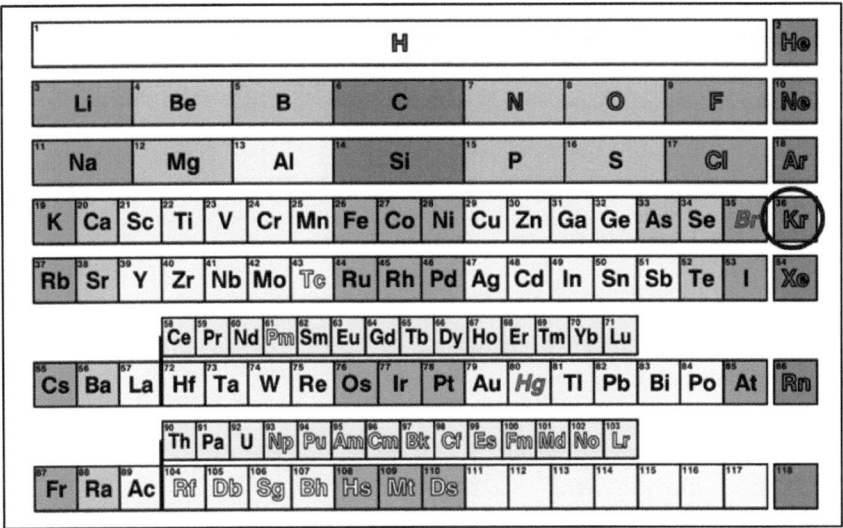

Figure 2.1 Krypton in the periodic table

it has since been discovered that they are relatively abundant on the Earth and in the universe. Helium is the second most plentiful element in the universe after hydrogen and is a product of nuclear fusion reactions that are the prime source of stellar energy. The other noble gases are likely to have been created by further nuclear condensation reactions deep within stars. As the atomic numbers increase, the gases become rarer. Neon, argon, krypton, and xenon were likely part of the original mass of gases that condensed to form the Earth. They are all present in the Earth's atmosphere forming five of the nine major constituents, which are constant when free air is sampled.

The main constituents of air

The following are the components of dry air:[2]

TABLE 2.1   The main constituents of air

Element	Volume by %	Weight by %	PPM (parts per million) by volume	Symbol of the element	Molecular weight of the element
Nitrogen	78.08	75.47	780790	N_2	28.01
Oxygen	20.95	23.20	209445	O_2	32.00
Argon	0.93	1.28	9339	Ar	39.95
Carbon Dioxide	0.040	0.062	404	CO_2	44.01
Neon	0.0018	0.0012	18.21	Ne	20.18
Helium	0.0005	0.00007	5.24	He	4.00
Krypton	0.0001	0.0003	1.14	Kr	83.80
Hydrogen	0.00005	Negligible	0.50	H_2	2.02
Xenon	8.7×10^{-6}	0.00004	0.087	Xe	131.30

Other components of air

Some other *components of air* are mentioned below:

- Sulfur dioxide *(SO2) – 1.0 ppm*
- Methane *(CH4) – 2.0 ppm*
- Nitrous oxide *(N2O) – 0.5 ppm*
- Ozone *(O3) – 0 to 0.07 ppm*
- Nitrogen dioxide *(NO2) – 0.02 ppm*
- Iodine *(I2) – 0.01 ppm*
- Carbon monoxide *(CO) – 0 to trace ppm*

One of the most well-known properties of noble gases is their ability to absorb and emit electromagnetic radiation, glowing when an electrical discharge is passed through any of the gases sealed in a glass tube. Pure neon produces a red-orange light; helium-argon forms an orange hue; neon-argon makes a deep lavender colour; krypton gives off bluish white light.

The noble gases are used as refrigerants due to their very low boiling and melting points.

History[2]

Krypton was discovered in 1898 in England by Sir William Ramsay (1852–1916), a Scottish born professor of chemistry at the University College, London and Morris W. Travers FRS (1872–1961). Having previously identified argon and isolated helium, Ramsay deduced that there had to be other gases present in the same group of the periodic table, and he set out with his student Travers, to discover what they were.

Together, they produced liquid air by cooling it to a low temperature. By using a process of fractional distillation, in which the liquid air is allowed to gradually warm and each of the gases boils at different temperature, they could be separated and identified.

During a period of three months, Ramsay and Travers managed to identify three new elements: neon, krypton, and xenon, a record that has not been broken. The noble gases were the last group of the periodic table to be discovered.

TABLE 2.2   Some of the properties of krypton

Atomic number	36
Atomic weight	83.80
Melting point	−157.2°C
Boiling point at 1 atm pressure	−153.35°C
Gas density at 0°C and 1 atm pressure g/liter	3.749
Liquid density at its boiling point, g/ml	2.413
Solubility in water at 20°C ml krypton per 1000g water at 1 atm partial pressure krypton	59.4
Valence	0, 2
Crystal structure	Face-centred cubic

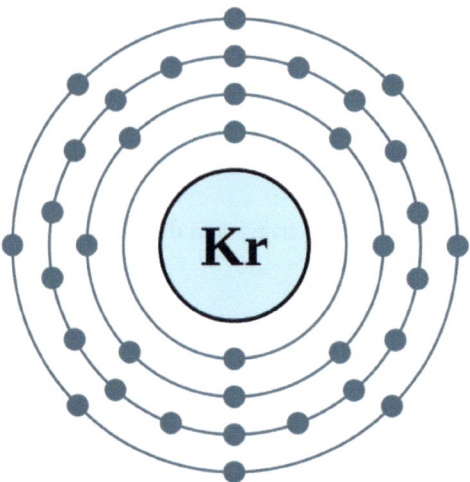

Figure 2.2 *Krypton atomic structure*

Properties[3]

Like all noble gases, krypton is colourless, odourless, and tasteless. It is nearly three times heavier than air. The outer shell of the krypton atom is filled with electrons (shell structure 2,8,18,8) giving it great stability (Figure 2.2). For this reason, its molecules are monoatomic and no compound of krypton is stable at room temperature. Krypton atoms are considered to have perfect spherical symmetry.

Isotopes[4]

Krypton has isotopes of every number from 74 to 95, six of these are stable 78, 80, 82, 83, 84, and 85.

There are also the following radioactive isotopes of krypton: 76, 77, 79, 81, 83 (metastable), 85, 87, 88, 89, 91, 92, 93, 94, 95 and 97. They are produced as byproducts of the nuclear fission of uranium and plutonium in nuclear reactors, and during reprocessing of spent fuel elements from nuclear reactors as well as in particle accelerators. The only radioactive isotope which is produced in more than traces and has quite a long half-life of 10.73 years is krypton-85, the others have half-lives of three hours or less.

Occurrence

The only commercial source of stable krypton is the air, although traces of krypton are found in minerals and meteorites. Krypton constitutes 1.14

parts per million by volume of the Earth's atmosphere. This krypton is almost entirely a mixture of the following isotopes, none of which are radioactive: 79 (0.35%), 80 (2.27%), 82 (11.56%), 83 (11.55%), 84 (56.9%), and 86 (17.37%).

A mixture of stable and radioactive isotopes of krypton is produced in nuclear reactors by the slow neutron fission of uranium.

It is estimated that about $2 \times 10^{-8}\%$ of the weight of the Earth is krypton. Krypton also occurs outside the Earth: the estimate is that there are 51 atoms of krypton for each 1,000,000 atoms of silicon in the visible universe.

Analytical methods

The principal modern methods of detecting and quantitatively determining the krypton content in gases are mass spectrometry and gas chromatography. The older method of detecting krypton makes use of its characteristic emission spectrum, obtained by passing a gas sample through an electric discharge tube and analysing the light with spectrometer.

Production[5]

Stable krypton is produced in air-separation plants. Air is liquefied and distilled; krypton and xenon remain with oxygen. The liquid oxygen is redistilled to concentrate the krypton and xenon from a few parts per million to a few percent. The rare gases are than absorbed from the liquid oxygen onto silica gel, desorbed, separated, and purified. Final production is carried out by passing the krypton over hot titanium metal, on which all except inert gas impurities are removed.

Radioactive krypton-85 is produced in nuclear reactors.

Uses[6]

Krypton's main use is as a filler gas in electric lamps, and specialised lights. A mixture of krypton-argon is used to fill fluorescent lamps.

As with xenon, krypton is becoming an increasingly important gas in the lighting sector. The car industry, for example, now offers headlights that work with krypton. This rare gas is also used as a filler gas in halogen bulbs, energy-saving bulbs, and gas discharge tubes in illuminated billboards. Replacing nitrogen/argon with krypton in halogen energy-saving lamps and fluorescent lamps increases bulb life and produces more effective lighting.

The inert nature of the noble gases makes them ideal as a filler of incandescent lamps. Despite the higher cost, krypton-filled lamps have two advantages: if the bulb is used at the same brightness, it will have very much longer life, or the brightness of the bulb can be increased. Krypton bulbs are therefore used in long-life bulbs, and when a small bright bulb is required as in projectors.

Most fluorescent tubes are filled with about half and half mixture of argon and krypton. Discharged ultraviolet radiation is converted to visible light by the phosphor coating on the tube wall.

Krypton is also used to fill electric-arc lamps. These lamps are capable of penetrating 300 metres of fog. Similar lamps are employed to mark airplane runways during bad visibility and at night, arranged in rows flashing 40 times a minute, each flash lasting 17 microseconds to avoid blinding the pilots. Krypton-filled bulbs are also employed in high-speed photography.

Radioactive krypton-85 has a number of applications in industry. Its advantages are relative cheapness, non-reactivity and easy detection of its radiation. Krypton-85 is used in detection of flaws in metal surfaces, leak testing of sealed containers, and measurement of thickness of materials such as metal and plastics.

Krypton is a key factor in energy-saving windows. It is used as a filler gas between insulated glass panes since its low thermal conductivity increases the effectiveness of insulation. 40% or more of all krypton produced worldwide is used for this purpose.

The international standard for the metre from 1960 to 1983 was defined in wavelengths of krypton light.

One metre is the length equal to 1,650,763.73 in vacuo of the radiation corresponding to the transition between energy levels 2p10 and 5d5 of the krypton atom.'[6]

Since 1983, one metre is defined as the distance travelled by light in a vacuum in 1/299,792,458 second.[7]

During the cold war, superpowers used the amount of krypton-85 detected in the atmosphere as a measure of nuclear activity undertaken by the opposing side.[3]

Reference

1   Air Composition and its Properties BYJU's Online Learning App. Available online at: https://tinyurl.com/dedh37bj (accessed 12 March, 2014).

2   Chemistry of Krypton. *Chemistry Libre Texts*. Available online at: http://tinyurl.com/2898kznd (accessed July 18, 2024).

3   Krypton. Chemical Periodic Table. *Chemicool.com.* 17 Oct. 2012. Web.
    7/18/2023. Available online at: http://tinyurl.com/y4sthfsz (accessed July 18,
    2023).

4   Krypton. *Royal Society of Chemistry.* Available online at. http://tinyurl.com/
    35tzfu44 (accessed July 18, 2023).

5   Krypton. *MadeHow.* Available online at: http://tinyurl.com/ykvaxt32 (accessed
    July 18, 2023).

6   Krypton. *Wikipedia.* Available online at: https://en.wikipedia.org/wiki/Krypton
    (accessed July 18, 2023).

7   Basic Units of Measurements. Available online at: http://tinyurl.com/39tx93yv
    (accessed July 18, 2023).

8   Gibb P. How is the speed of light measured? *The Original Usenet Physics FAQ*
    (1997). Available online at: http://tinyurl.com/y7tu29w3 (accessed July 18,
    2023).

3

KRYPTON MOTHER TINCTURE

Krypton was prepared and potentised at Helios Pharmacy in Tunbridge Wells, UK as follows:

Analytic grade 99.998% krypton gas was bubbled through purified water for 20 minutes. Krypton's solubility in water is 0.16g in 100ml = 1.6×10^{-4}.

This aqueous solution was considered to be 2c.

3c was prepared in 50% BP ethanol.

The 4c potency and above were made with 90% ethanol following the Hahnemannian method using 10 succussions at each step.

4

KRYPTON 12C:
PHYSICAL AFFINITIES

The main affinities of the proving are heart, head, eyes, chest and respiration, back, extremities, vertigo, face, skin, throat.

It takes much clinical experience with a remedy to find out its most prominent affinities. Based on the cases I and colleagues have seen, I have highlighted the important aspects of Krypton with the most prominent in CAPS.

BACK and SHOULDER pain. HEART, blood and circulation. Head and headaches (after apoplexy), FOREHEAD (Frontal lobe, Third Eye), vertigo, impetigo, cold sores, flus and upper respiratory infections, DIFFICULT BREATHING, asthma, cough, neck ache, REPETITIVE SPRAINS and STRAINS. Work-related repetitive sprain injury, sleeplessness.

For more details refer to the cases in Chapter 13.

5

KRYPTON 30C: GENERALITIES

The following is a discussion of Krypton's generalities and most prominent particular symptoms.

Sensation of being very tall, dreams and images of elongated people like Giacometti statues. Sensation of elongation or distortion of body parts. Nose, jaw, and lip feel elongated. Opposing this is a need to curl up completely like a fossil. Sensation of sliding downwards, accompanied with despair. Low energy, faintness, lethargy, tiredness, oppression, heavy feeling, better occupation. Sensation of 'walking through treacle', as if 'body going into necrosis'. Low sexual energy. Stiffness with desire to stretch. Tendency to put on weight. Waking too early or too late. Awkward and clumsy.

Sensation of heat and hot flushes. Rushing of blood to head. Desire and amelioration from cool fresh air. Sensation of coldness, and skin feels cold to the touch. Cold and heat alternating.

Intense desire for chocolate and hot chocolate drinks. Desire organic dark chocolate due to tiredness. Desire alcohol, brandy, bread, garlic, miso, olives, potatoes, tahini, salmon, sweets, cold water. Aversion to meat, tobacco and chocolate.

Aggravation from the new and full moon and lack of sun. Periodicity, 24 hours and monthly. Better on waking.

Sensation as from a magnet or radiation. Sensation of water trickling down the head. A variety of headaches, especially pressing. Pain and tension in the skull. Vertigo can be quite severe, with aggravation on motion and nausea, worse in the afternoon. Sensation of a foreign body in the eye, tired eyes, twitching of eyelids. Seeing colours and auras. Ears hot and red. Sharp pains in the ears. Hot flashes on face. Constriction and tightness of chest. Difficult respiration and cough. Squeezing and tightness of heart with rapid pulse. Stiffness and pain of neck. Dislocation of back with sensation of spine separating and moving in two different directions. Pain in lower back as if labour pain with bearing down sensation. Sciatica. Tendency to burn fingers. Pain in index finger.

6

KRYPTON 200C:
EMOTIONAL ESSENCE

The clever men at Oxford
Know all that there is to be knowed.
But they none of them know one half as much
As intelligent Mr Toad!

Kenneth Grahame[1]

Cryptic Krypton is the most complex remedy in the materia medica, full of riddles, maths, geometry, and codes. It is a remedy of intellect, representing the birth of mankind's frontal lobe, the flowering of knowledge with its ability to measure, compare, analyse, and drive itself crazy. Krypton is the clockmaker, the one who cuts time into units and makes it go round in circles. He is the Asperger mathematician, the mapmaker, the physicist, the computer programmer, the bored office worker, the code creator, and the code breaker.

Krypton presents a clear and strong picture and is one of the frequently prescribed remedies of my Dynamis provings. Once its essential nature is grasped, it cannot be missed or replaced, though it is a multifaceted and complex remedy which is certain to have many more clinical aspects then I have used so far. I must warn you, that by its very nature, Krypton can be the most fascinating of remedies but at the same time most tedious.

Naturally Krypton shares some of the common noble gas themes, such as desire for cleanliness, tidiness, and truth, as well as their opposites: scruffiness and concealment. The noble tendency to avoid interacting with others manifests in a sense of disconnection. This disconnection may be due to an emotional trauma such as disappointed love affairs and broken hearts.

Yet Krypton has its own unique nature that distinguishes it from the other nobles. Perhaps the most common theme is of boredom and frustration at work. The feeling is of tedious repetition, an uninspired monotonous cycle in which the same things occur day in and day out, with a desire to get off the treadmill. This often relates to tiresome mental work, where the spark of creativity is lacking. Patients might feel like slaves to the system, longing for freedom or lost childhood fun. They may compensate with spiritual practices.

Krypton marks the descent into irreversible and desperate chronic disease, where time increases rather than solves pathology. The remedy relates to the word 'chronic' (from Greek *khronikos* "of time, concerning time"). Time is an essential aspect of Krypton, especially when it becomes cyclical and repetitive; the patient is a prisoner of his own rhythms. The converse is also true in this remedy. When our hearts are aligned with the Source, they beat to the tempo of the universe rather than to their own rhythm. In this case, as with the other noble gases, Krypton has a spiritual aspect, a sense of continuum and a blissful connection to the Divine.

The divine sense of Krypton is quite different from that of Helium, Neon or Argon. This is not the soul in its incarnation, the blissful newborn baby, or the playful youth. The spirituality of Krypton is intellectual and relates to esoteric systems of knowledge and the nature of the 'mind'. These interests may include Egyptology, Buddhism (especially Tibetan), karma, astronomy, physics, or mathematics. One patient had a great interest in ancient Mexican cultures, Mayan or Aztec. Other manifestations of this intellectual tendency are an affinity for riddles, cryptograms, numbers, codes, hieroglyphics, logic and mathematical puzzles, and computer programming. Chronos and its Latin analog Saturn are related to darkness, the hidden, and the cave. This is where Krypton becomes Cryptic. The Krypton patient is often quite cerebral, and logic overrides the heart. Just studying and thinking about the remedy Krypton is a mental effort. It is a code wrapped in an enigma combined with a cypher. My brain got so tired from working on this book I had to take a seven-year break before resuming. Mental exertion is a big feature of this remedy.

Krypton seems to have an affinity to computers and computer programmers, with a speciality in losing data. Many a hard drive has crashed while working on this remedy, and I had to recover the data numerous times. Provings were jumbled, cases lost. It seems fitting that I cannot find any 'Intellect' symptoms in this proving, i.e. confusion, concentration or memory. Either they were all lost or none were noticed in the proving. I am fairly sure other sections went missing in cyberspace.

When people hear of the remedy Krypton, their first association is often Superman. Of all the 20th century comic heroes, Superman is undoubtedly the most powerful and noble. Superman is an extra-terrestrial who is sent from the planet Krypton, and his superpowers are only susceptible to Kryptonite from his planet. Does Superman relate to this remedy? There are several similarities between the picture of Krypton and everyone's favourite superhero. While he is totally committed to doing good on this planet, his emotional world and love life are not very successful. High IQ, low EQ (emotional intelligence).

Krypton has a strong connection to extra-terrestrial beings, UFO's, the sky, planets, stars and the moon. It seems that Krypton echoes Neon's love and yearning for the heavens. Krypton has an attraction to sky burials, where the dead are laid on a platform, to be eaten by the birds and recycled to the heavens.

Krypton has a strong desire for chocolate. Before the proving, I never realised how many chocolate names were galactic.

Dream of names of chocolate brands – Mars, Galaxy, Milky Way, Aero, Ripple, Swirl, and I liked After-Eight.

One prover was extremely angry with me for 'causing' her to re-upholster a sofa with pictures of star signs on it. She had not noticed what they were, as the signs were upside down; she thought they were hieroglyphics. Upside down writing, mirror writing, astrology and hieroglyphs are all typical aspects of this remedy.

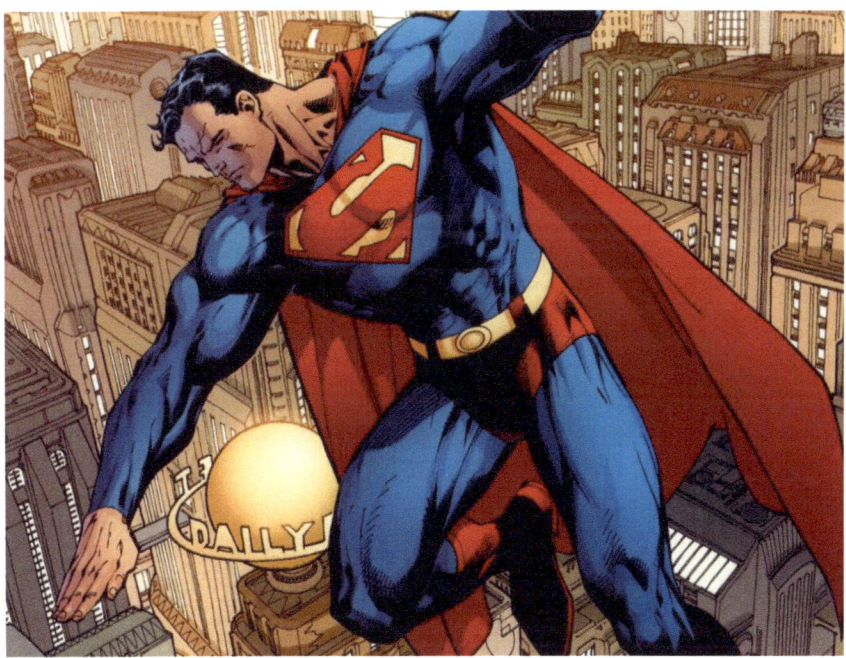

Figure 6.1 Superman, from the planet Krypton, exemplifies various characteristics found in the Krypton proving. See Chapter 15.

Like Superman, patients needing this remedy may be heroic, or dream of it. Yet this remedy also depicts the mundane existence of superman's alter ego, the timid and boring journalist Clark Kent. Krypton also echoes the sad story of Christopher Reeves, the actor famous for his film role as Superman. Following an accident, Reeves became paralysed from the head down, remaining with a keen intellect but a useless body.

When it comes to sorting out humanity's problems, Superman has one unique power: Though it is strictly forbidden, he is able to reverse the flow of time by flying around the earth and changing the direction of its rotation. And herein lies one of the secrets of this remedy: In which direction are we and our timescale rotating, and in fact, why are we rotating at all?

Reference

1   Grahame K. The Song of Mr Toad. In: *The Wind in the Willows* (1908). Book available online at http://tinyurl.com/4v24djut (Quote available online at: http://tinyurl.com/2p8mjvxf (accessed January 29, 2024.))

7

1M: HIGHER EMOTIONAL THEMES

Ticking away the moments that make up a dull day
You fritter and waste the hours in an offhand way.
Kicking around on a piece of ground in your hometown
Waiting for someone or something to show you the way.

Pink Floyd[1]

The following are the main mental and emotional themes of Krypton in more detail, each with a few examples from the proving. At the end of the chapter, we will try to construct a meaningful picture.

Mental emotional themes

Clean/dirty

Like the other noble gases Krypton has perfectionist tendencies, which may manifest in cleaning, washing and organising – activities which they enjoy. Yet they may also look extremely scruffy and unkempt. I have seen several Krypton cases who previously received Sulphur due to their shabby and dirty clothes combined with the intellectual theorizing nature.

I cleaned every surface and every inch of the kitchen! Felt great satisfaction through achievement at the end of it.
Very strong urge to wash the bedding. Everything must be clean.
Desire to tidy the flat. My mood improves while doing it.
I'm streamlining my life. I feel so organized.
Cleanliness, angry about clothes being spoiled and dirtied.
I went out with dirty clothes and hair. I haven't worn make-up for 2 days. I don't care what I look like.
I went to work with dirty clothes. My cardigan was so filthy that I had to take it off and hide it.

Superhero and animal clothes

While there is no direct reference to Superman in the proving, the super-person's tendency to wear underwear over clothes may be seen in the following humorous occurrence:

Tried to put my bra on over my blouse in the car.

One prover felt that she was:

Travelling at 300,000 km per second

Krypton may have a peculiar desire to dress in leopard skin clothes. This may indicate a feeling of having a powerful animal force. One patient who responded very well to Krypton had a childhood fantasy of being Tarzan.

In a shop, I noticed a leopard-skin swimsuit and I really wanted to buy it. I had a strong desire to wear it. Previously I would never have considered wearing such a swimsuit.

Strongly attracted to mock leopard skin. Bought hat and gloves and bag. Wanted the strength of the animal prints.

Attraction to loud animal skin clothes.

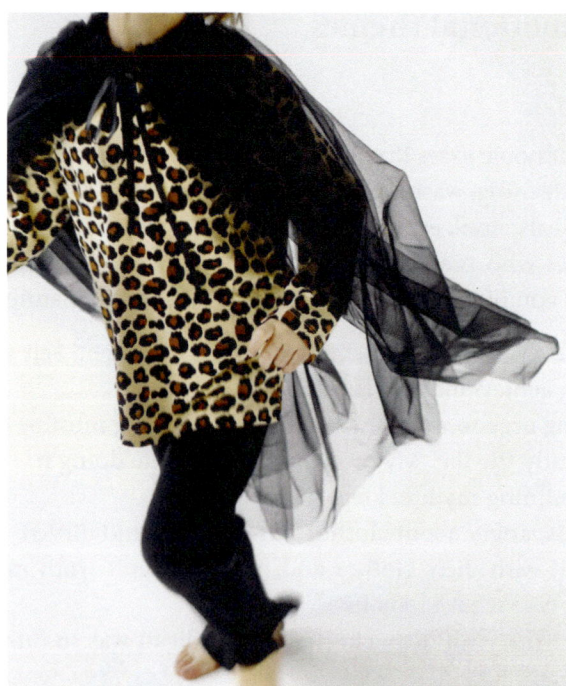

Figure 7.1 Leopard clothing

Sky

From the Krypton point of view, people come from the sky and should return to the sky. (Notice echoes of Neon, Noble 2 in Krypton, Noble 4.)

The sky – clouds and stars- seems so close, I could almost touch it if I stretch my arm.

On passing a cemetery, thought they weren't a good idea – felt sky burials were much more appropriate. The sky is doubly important to me. Pleased that there is more sky than anything.

On the radio they were talking about Christ from cross to grave to sky – sky burials.

My enthusiasm to skydive has become much more intense.

Moon

While looking at the moon, thoughts come into my mind: "I love it", "I want to reach the moon".

The moon is so full, strong and clear. Have never seen it so enormous. I try to look at it whenever possible.

I felt the moon belonged to me, like in "The Little Prince". It was like parting with a lover you know so intimately, and now have to share with others.

Stars

Twinkle, twinkle, little star.
How I wonder what you are.

A&J Taylor[2]

Dream of a falling star.

Seeing star images all around me. All I want to do is buy star objects. I'm in love with stars.

Before falling asleep, I moved to **align myself directly** with the stars through the sky window in my room. I joined the stars as I fell asleep. (JS – Compare Neon)

Dream of names of chocolate brands – Mars, Galaxy, Milky Way, Aero, Ripple, Swirl.

Time is not equal and there are still points for entering the Stargates.

Discovered that the patterns on the newly covered sofa were Star signs. When we bought the material I thought they were just hieroglyphics or random patterns, but it turned out they were upside down Star signs.

Have been thinking about the symbolism of stars. The Seal of Solomon; spirit and matter meeting.

Found a wonderful pair of silvery star earrings.

Alien

I'm sure the universe is full of intelligent life.
It's just been too intelligent to come here.

Arthur C. Clarke[3]

Superman is not the only alien to descend from the stars that relates to Krypton. Krypton has a strong affinity to UFO's and extraterrestrials.

I suddenly felt totally alien like from another planet.

Dream of being a star child.

I'm in a strange city. It is some kind of meeting. There are people of different nationalities and races including aliens. Nobody quite knows what is going on. Things are not what they seem. (JS – Compare Crypto-coccus, also saying 'things are not what they seem'.)

Dream, I look up at the night sky, and I see several shooting stars. I get excited and tell people who are with me to look up. The shooting stars are redder than normal, like sparks in a fire. As the sky brightens at dawn, I realize that the sparks are coming from a dark moving sphere like a tail of a comet. As the sphere gets closer and lower, I notice spheres coming from all directions to surround one main sphere. Gradually they all descend and disappear over the horizon. I stand transfixed and shocked as I realise that I have seen the landing of a UFO.

Astronomy and numbers

Astronomy has a relationship with numbers and mathematics, and Krypton patients love both. The proving of Krypton brought forth many references to astronomy, numbers and mathematical expressions. The following are some examples. In a later chapter we will examine the individual meaning of these peculiar expressions. Meanwhile note the number 36 and its components.

Red giants are cooler and the blue much hotter. The white were more compressed and compact. Thoughts about how the sun is 8 minutes away, but our other nearest star is *Proxima centauri*. I felt I was travelling at 300,000 km per second.

Quasars – blue and compact emit a very strong radio wave, stronger than is possible. It's to do with us not understanding why there is 30 something % more matter in the universe than we can calculate.

Celestial equators 90 degrees. Plus it in the North and minus it in the South. A square on the equator is a point on the pole.

Dream that Keppler and Newton were talking about the 12 tribes and 12 pearls, then the fact that 12 was 3×4 and 3 was the first wholly odd number and 4 the first even. Then they were discussing how no-one yet can draw a perfect heptagon, because it has not yet been revealed. The reason we can't draw it is because it is dynamic and not static. Talking about the 5th dimension not yet created.

2H atoms collide to make heavy hydrogen. A third H atom makes HE3 beryllium when they separate again. Another He makes He4 + 2H, released as stable helium, very fast, and timeless.

In my mind's eye, I was seeing magic squares and how our sun is 6×6 which is 36, and Venus is 7×7.

Woke after a dream. Fish were multiplying – now there were 139, or were there 136?

Only seeing male patients today – ages 4, 8, 12 and 36. A series.

$E = M(O)exp(-AT)$ *

Codes

It is one of the remarkable 'synchronicities' that unite chemistry, linguistics and provings that the name *krypton* was chosen for element 36. Every 100 liters of liquid air contains about one-tenth of a milliliter of krypton, just one drop. So, Ramsay and Travers – although they didn't know it – were looking for one drop of krypton in 100 liters of liquid air. Therefore they named the scarce element krypton.

Krypton comes from the Greek *kryptos* (The Hidden One), or *krypte* short for *krypte kamara* (hidden vault). The related word crypt, originating from the Latin *crypta* or the Greek *kryptē* means concealed. Cryptic means hidden, secret, occult, mystical, encoded. In this context it is strange to see the several similarities between Krypton and Cryptococcus neoformans, though the latter is much more poisonous and psychedelic. Both remedies tell: Things are not what they seem; hence code.

In architecture a crypt is a stone chamber or vault often beneath the floor of a church containing sarcophagi, coffins or relics. In anatomy crypts are cavities or narrow pouches formed by a folding back or turning inside out of tissues within a larger structure.

True to its name, Krypton loves codes and riddles. I have found clinically that Krypton patients love mathematical puzzles or code games. I began writing *Dynamic Materia Medica: Syphilis*[4] during the Krypton proving. I was obsessed with concealing the inner secrets, so that the final book was over-encoded and I had to publish a second edition with commentary. Many Krypton symptoms appear to be in code form, and can be understood in a variety of ways. In a later chapter, we will attempt to crack some of these codes. Here are some examples:

Dream there was an entry code to the building with numbers beginning 63.

There was a joke when I woke: Four cons = it was cryptic. Con cave or was the cave a con? A "C" is a quarter of an "8". Dismember the * and you get four C's.

Dreams of crypts and things being cryptic and Coptic, of Egypt and Osiris. Four faces, but five lines. It was about either to serve, preserve, or conserve.

In my mind's eye, I was seeing magic squares and how our sun is 6×6 which is 36, and Venus is 7×7.

Mirror

One of the most ancient forms of coding was mirror writing, which appears prominently in the proving.

PHAT! A word used to bring a corpse back to life. Also used backwards TAHP. It is not to be said aloud, so you encode it.

I was witnessing the birth of letters, seeing them coming into being in English and Hebrew. Hebrew starts at the back of the book.

Passed through Oldhill, for which the sign read Hold Ill (holding on to being ill – the security of having symptoms) and at Snow Hill, the sign reads Now Hills.

Writing right to left.

On own now, now own one, no own now, own one/won, we won.

The Rabbi says it's OK if I have an H in my name. H and A are the same in mirror image.

Amy also spells Yam and May if you change the letters around.

Dream there was an entry code to the building with numbers beginning 63.

(JS – note the mirror writing of 63)

Truth

Like the other nobles, Krypton relates strongly to the truth, as opposed to being encrypted.

The blind-spot in the eye exists for the mind to see the truth.

Seeing things as they are, absolute state – knowing that the true nature of the mind is the true nature of everything.

Time

> *Time is the substance I am made of. Time is a river which sweeps me along, but I am the river; it is a tiger which destroys me, but I am the tiger; it is a fire which consumes me, but I am the fire.*
>
> *straight line begins to curl*
>
> Jorge Luis Borges[5]

In my personal life I am usually late, about 15 minutes overtime by default. During the proving, I was either early or exactly on time, which was quite unusual. When I was teaching in Ireland during the proving, the clocks changed to summertime. I arrived one hour early while the students, in true Irish fashion, were one hour late. I waited for two hours. Since the proving I have changed my attitude and prefer to be on time or early.

As you will later see, TIME in all its variations is one of the most important aspects of Krypton. Krypton seems to be able to affect time in any which way. Provers were either floating in the present, traveling back and forth in time, arriving late, being uncharacteristically punctual, or recycling time. Here is an abbreviated collection of several provers' expressions 'As If One Person' (A.I.O.P).

How flexible time is. Time is not equal. The concept of time has changed. It feels more as a continuum present rather than in compartments of before, past, later. I went through the ages of time. Not really in touch with time, not really knowing what time it was. It was as if time wasn't really existing. Conscious of the present moment, continuum present. I wish I could go back in time. Arrived one hour early. Losing sense of time and end up being late for appointments. Difficult to calculate time. I feel in sync with the universe.

Computer

Computers make it easier to do a lot of things, but most of the things they make it easier to do don't need to be done.

Andy Rooney[6]

No one ever said on their deathbed, 'Gee, I wish I had spent more time alone with my computer'.

Danielle Berry[7]

Krypton loves computers, is aggravated by computers, and crashes computers. I recall many times when the Krypton proving data was lost with the death of someone's unfortunate hard drive. Most likely, some of the proving symptoms will never be recovered. Being an intellectual remedy, Krypton relates to those who use computers too much, such as analysts, programmers, people who work with code. Patients can also behave a bit like computers.

I sold my computer today. It was constantly breaking down on me, God, I hope it will work for the new owner!

I am seeking distraction from mental work by looking at my databases a long time.

My computer keeps crashing, it angers me.

Computer breakdown, associated with a forsaken feeling. Feeling that some giant force took over my electrical equipment.

I felt irritated after sitting in front of the big computer screen. It felt as if the computer had interfered and broken the electro-magnetic field of the remedy.

The last symptom is reminiscent of a physical symptom some provers experienced, a sensation of a magnet on various body parts. Perhaps Krypton patients emit a magnetic energy which crashes their hard drives.

Measuring

I was stretching upwards. I normally have a delusion 'tall' but I actually said I was 36 hands. Do you know how they measure horses, in hands?

The element krypton is used for precise measuring, and likewise the Krypton nature may be precise and perfectionist. In the past the krypton isotope was used for measuring the length of the meter.

The relative quantities of krypton versus hydrogen can be used by astronomers to measure how much nucleosynthesis (element formation) has taken place in any region of interstellar space.

Krypton absorption at ~77°K is considered the standard and most accurate method for surface area measurements of materials with very low surface area. The measurements are in nano-meters. Krypton isotherms are used to measure the specific surface area, pore diameter, pore size distribution, and pore volume of thin, mesoporous silica films. These films have applications in many electronic fields, e.g. sensors.

During the cold war, superpowers used the amount of krypton-85 detected in the atmosphere as a measure of nuclear activity undertaken by the opposing side.

Here is a proving thought from Silvie (The proving was double blind):

I woke up wondering what Krypton Tuning was.

Crypton was the trade name one of the first electronic engine tuning systems in the early 1960's, used for tuning engines. Hence the name "Crypton Tuning". Similar equipment was manufactured by several companies, but Crypton was the market leader so people picked up on the name. This system is now obsolete. It is not relevant to modern cars, rather for old Cortinas and Escorts.

Many of the Krypton measuring systems mentioned above are now out of date, replaced by elements such as caesium or by light years. Modern measurement requires ultra-precise instruments relating to the 5th, 6th and 7th periods. The 4th period is now obsolete for measuring.

Head off

Finally, we find a curious reference to the Krypton head being chopped off. Obviously, this is symbolic of having no intellect. Or perhaps going around in circles.

Dream of a female probation officer without her head.

When lying in bed, a sudden delusion of a guillotine falling down from the roof cutting my head off.

The word 'beheaded' came up.

Very strange dream as it seemed that the intellect part of myself detached from someone powerful ... the inner centre was undisturbed.

The hanged man on the Tarot cards. I don't want to talk to anyone at all, only patients at work. I have gone all hermetic.

Conclusion – bringing it all together

I have tried 99 times and have failed, but on the 100th time came success.

Albert Einstein[8]

We have studied several aspects of Krypton's mental picture. We have seen Krypton's clean and highly organized disposition, and its opposite scruffiness. This perfectionism is related to a desire to tell the truth, both common features in the perfectly-formed complete nobles. The opposing side is concealing the truth behind codes and mirror writing. Clean and dirty, truth and code are contradictory aspects of the Krypton nature.

Consider this: Krypton is an extremely intellectual remedy, though its desire to wear leopard skin reveals something of its opposite, instinctive animal side. The word 'consider' means to think carefully about something, to reflect, to ponder a problem. Its etymological root is 'to look at the stars'. We have seen Krypton's desire to look to the moon, stars and planets, to embrace UFO's and aliens which descend from the sky, and to return the dead to the sky though sky burials. We know the mythology of Superman, the noble extraterrestrial from the distant planet Krypton.

Astronomy, which Krypton is attracted to, is powered by numbers, and numbers relate to code. Codes are the driving force behind computers, as in computer coding. Computers depend on the accurate rhythm of their beating heart, the CPU (central processing unit). A CPU's time keeping must be extremely precise, measured in billions of oscillations per second. Time is a major factor in Krypton. Time relates to the stars; it is by the cycle of sun, moon, planets and constellations that we measure its passage. Krypton is precise in measuring both distance and time, and for this measurement we need an exacting intellect. With its head cut off, the Krypton intellect separates from its heart. We find an exacting computer-like, number-measuring intellect residing in a brain disconnected from heart and alienated from animal instinct. This pure intellect seeks the direct, dry truth, without the ability to soften it with feeling. And so, we come full circle. But to break this circle, to crack the Kryptic code, we must spiral up the scale to a higher potency of perception.

Negative emotional themes

Watch out for intellect,
because it knows so much it knows nothing
and leaves you hanging upside down,
mouthing knowledge as your heart
falls out of your mouth.

Anne Sexton[9]

Training session at work, made me think around separating thoughts from feelings.

In the previous section, we examined some mental aspects of Krypton. By mental, I refer to the intellect, which in Krypton appears to be over-functioning, revolving around codes, numbers, computers, and astro-nomical considerations. By themselves, these characteristics would not be pathological, but for the fact that the intense intellect overrides and suppresses emotions. This leaves a horrible sense of disconnection, one which my wife (then girlfriend) and I were unfortunate enough to experi-ence during the proving. Here is the summary of what we felt for those few months. It was as if we had descended from the lofty height of love to the valley of detachment.

Disconnected

We as a couple feel that through the proving we have lost the deep **heart-love** connection that we have felt for two years, and although we realise and know intellectually that we love each other it seems to come from a different place, more from the intellect or forehead or, on the other hand, from a sexual connection. But the **heart** feels far away, difficult to reach. As if we are sliding helplessly down from lofty mountain of love and there is nothing we can do about it. This is scaring us.

Yet on the level of cerebral intellect, we feel more powerful and positive, more able to achieve.

A continuous disconnection that leaves only the hopeless possibility of despair and dreariness with little possibility of ever getting it right or returning to our former blissful state. A **heart**less, hopeless feeling.

Disconnected. I know that I love my boyfriend, but I know it intellectu-ally, my **heart** doesn't feel it. I'm not loving him totally from the **heart** as I was before.

I realised that I had lost connection to God.

I never knew what it is like not to be connected to God. I never knew I was connected before.

Dis-membered, Dis-connection

The disconnection in Krypton is not only spiritual and emotional. There is a prominent theme of being *dismembered*, or cut into pieces.

There was a TV program of somebody's daughter being dismembered and fed to alligators.

Feels as if upper torso is disconnected. Left and right across the upper part of my heart, and front and back at the lower.

Member means being a part of the body or a part of a group. We need to remember that we are dismembered – cut off from the one – the love, we are being beckoned.

We believe our mind is separate from the universal mind.

Dream that I was asked about joints, which joints were disjointed and which double jointed.

On the walls at Karnak are dismembered hands and penises.

Sensation of being in 14 parts, each disconnected from the others, with penis having fallen off. Osiris was an Egyptian, he was cut into 14 pieces, the torso is quartered.

Kronos – emasculated father of Uranus. (JS – It was the opposite: Uranus was the father of Kronos the father of Zeus. But this is what the proving says. Mirror writing?)

Kronos (Cronus) was the King of the Titans and the god of time, in particular **time when viewed as a destructive, all-devouring force**. He ruled the cosmos during the Golden Age after castrating and deposing his father Ouranos (Uranus, Sky). In fear of a prophecy that he would in turn be overthrown by his own son, Kronos swallowed each of his children as they were born.[5,10]

Heart

Note that in some of the symptoms above I have emphasised the word *heart*. Krypton, the fourth noble, relates to the fourth chakra – the heart chakra. It is here that the disconnection is felt. All mind, no heart.

A friend was digging and pulling at my ribs – she wanted to show my heart. She said your heart is holding onto your memories.

Thoughts about the heart. Sensation of heart beating like a drum.

Feels as if upper torso is disconnected. Left and right across the upper part of my heart.

Karma is like a boomerang, and maybe a change of mind but now a change of heart.

And the opposite expectation that proves the rule:

This is given to us, no mind all heart, freely given.

The ratio of the symptoms above reminds me of the five provers who guessed that the proving remedy was Krypton. Four from the mind, and one from the heart.

Work

> *Choose a job you love, and you will never have to work*
> *a day in your life.*
>
> Anonymous[11]

> *The brain is a wonderful organ; it starts working the moment you*
> *get up in the morning and does not stop until you get into the office.*
>
> Robert Frost[12]

Krypton concludes the fourth period of the periodic table. In homoeo-pathic thinking, this period has a well-known association with profession and work. The problem with Krypton is that work is devoid of passion, there is no heart in it, it is a job rather than a vocation. Similar to the separation from the heart we saw above, Krypton's work is disconnected from its mission, leaving a resentful lack of motivation. They go to work because they have to, and it becomes a repetitive daily grind, a treadmill which they long to get off of. The office is a prison. The following are symptoms from different provers, arranged As If One Person (AIOP):

Disgruntled, irritable as soon as I walk into my office. I'm extremely irritated that I've got to do work that is not related to mine. Everything seems slowed down and have difficulty concentrating. Simple tasks like making the bed are impossible to complete. Overwhelmed with things I have to do but can't get organized to do any of it. Lack of motivation. Feeling of ambivalence at lack of motivation and feel serene inside. Embarking on another unnecessary task. Oh how can I be really free?!

Homoeopathic Haikus (JS)[1]

Night falls
a gentle wind blows.
I open my laptop

                    Sighing
                    I lean back.
                    who is this patient?

Finding the remedy
I rest my case.
The telephone rings

---

[1] Haiku is a short unrhymed poetic form that first appeared in Japanese literature in the 17th Century.

Boredom

He who seeks rest finds boredom. He who seeks work finds rest.

Dylan Thomas[13]

Boredom: the desire for desires.

Leo Tolstoy[14]

The Krypton lack of passion inevitably leads to boredom. A.I.O.P:
Nothing happens. I'm so bored. I behave in a more detached way. I don't want to do anything. Totally disinterested. Nothing excites me. I'm bored with everything. Life doesn't interest me.

Guilt, embarrassment, shame, failure
The guilt and shame of Krypton often arise from not measuring up to their perfect noble standard. AIOP:

Felt clever and crafty, but anxious and guilty, dishonest, a cheat. Feel embarrassment and shame about my emotions, if only I could not be constantly observing or caring who and how I am. Able to name an emotion never named before: Shame. Shame that I'm not perfect, that I make mistakes. Feel crushed inside when I make a mistake. Feel shame about expressing/having emotions. If only I didn't feel the fear of failure, the fear of standing up in front of others and looking or feeling stupid. I want to be perfect now, without practicing on real people and possibly failing.

Worthless
Dream had intercourse with a man for the first time, no passion on his part, I wondered if I was not as sexy as I used to be. Wondered if I would get pregnant or catch something from him, as he was a playboy. He was covered in acne on chest and arms.

Dream: A taxi driver was going to collect us from the airport. Wondered why we weren't collected in a limo. We're not special enough, not worth it.

Sleeplessness with feelings of humiliation and self-reproach, weeping all night to unfreeze my being and trying to reunite all the shredded bits with my centre.

Danger
Dream I am followed by three or four young men in a car. Kidnapped and drugged, but not to death, in spite of their efforts, I managed to escape. I later see them driving in my neighborhood and realise they are looking for me. Again, an acute sense of danger, "run for your life", no one to turn to.

Dream: My ex-boyfriend is after me, wants to do me bodily harm, and just when he's about to hurt me, three girls enter the ladies' toilet where I tried to hide from him. He can't attack me in their presence, but before he leaves he says silently: "You won't get away next time".

Conclusion

Run, rabbit run.
Dig that hole, forget the sun,
And when at last the work is done
Don't sit down it's time to dig another one

Pink Floyd[1]

What a difference between miserable Krypton and the happy Argon! While Argon, at its positive peak, dances the magic garden of childhood, the joys of youth and carefree teenage love, Krypton is stuck in the office with a computer and a dead relationship, disconnected from love and purpose, repeating the same task over and over again. This difference was very apparent during the proving, as I proved Argon and Krypton simultaneously in two different groups. The first group glowed with ease of flow, while the second bore the heavy burden of intellect devoid of passion.

That is the difference between the magic age of 18 and its tragic double, 36 – provided we lose the thread -the thread running from our Helium's soul mission through Neon's baby bliss and into Argon's passion of youth. If we cannot retain this connection, work becomes a lifelong prison sentence; clocking in and clocking out of the office, chained to a family and mortgage. When time has no heart to beat its rhythm, it becomes bland. Intellectual perfectionism rebukes the weaker emotions, resulting in a sense of disconnection, guilt, shame, failure, worthlessness and ultimately a danger to our lives.

Saw a movie 'LA Confidential' last night. It really irritated me. What a cold movie without any emotions. Just observation, no emotions, like a cartoon. It made me upset.

This is where we return to the idea of aliens. While Krypton suits some patients who claim to see or dream of UFO's, this is not the main issue. If we translate the idea of aliens to our internal landscape, we see how Krypton may be alienated from itself. We like to think of aliens as being more intelligent than we are. And they probably are, given that they made it all the way across the universe to our planet. Krypton may be hyper-intelligent, but this binary intelligence floats above, separated from the heart, disconnected from animal instinct and intuition. Extraterrestrial versus Neanderthal.

References

1 Pink Floyd. *Breathe* from the album *Dark Side of the Moon*. Harvest Records, 1973). Lyric available online at: http://tinyurl.com/mrxaju86 (accessed January 16, 2024).

2 Taylor A, Taylor J. *The Star, 1806*. Quote from lyrics available online at: http://tinyurl.com/y4vjanda (accessed January 10, 2024).

3 Clarke AC. *AZ Quotes*. Available online at: www.azquotes.com/quote/651327 (accessed July, 1823).

4 Sherr J. *Dynamic Materia Medica: Syphilis* (2nd edn, reprint). Glasgow: Saltire Books, 2021.

5 Borges JL. (ed: Irby JL). In: *Labyrinths: Selected Stories & Other Writings*. London: Pinguin Modern Classics, 2000. Quote available online at: http://tinyurl.com/2p9jzjz4 (accessed July 18, 2023).

6 Rooney A. *Brainy Quote*. Available online at: http://tinyurl.com/2bahpkva (accessed July 18, 2023).

7 Berry D. *Brainy Quote*. Available online at: http://tinyurl.com/3audxe7a (accessed July 18, 2023).

8 Einstein A. *Quotefancy*. Available online: http://tinyurl.com/yxjf88un (accessed July 18, 2023).

9 Sexton A. Admonitions to a Special Person. In: *The Complete Poems*. Bost9onMA: Houghton Mifflin, 1981.

10 Kronos. *Greek Mythology*, Available online at: http://tinyurl.com/56z298k7 (accessed July 17, 2023).

11 Anonymous. *Quote Investigator*. Available online at: http://tinyurl.com/m-w76sjp5 (accessed July 18, 2023).

12 Frost R. *Robert Frost quotes*. Available online at: http://tinyurl.com/34awtyz6 (accessed July 18, 2023).

13 Thomas D. *Dylan Thomas Quotes*. Available online at: http://tinyurl.com/3c8c989d (accessed July 18, 2023).

14 Tolstoy L. *Leo Tolstoy Quotes*. Available online at: http://tinyurl.com/2w547mbn (accessed July 18, 2023).

8

KRYPTON 10M:
SPIRITUAL THEMES

But beyond the mind, beyond our thoughts, there is something we call the 'nature of the mind', the mind's true condition, which is beyond all limits. If it is beyond the mind, though, how can we approach an understanding of it?
Chogyal Namkhai Nor[1]

Gravitation is not responsible for people falling in love.
Albert Einstein[2]

Spirituality

Transcending the mental and emotional level we arrive at the spiritual aspects of Krypton. Like its predecessors Helium, Neon and Argon, Krypton is highly connected to the spiritual world. Due to their vertical alignment, the nobles are placed on different rungs of the upright ladder to heaven. Each noble expresses its unique level of truth and spirituality, of being in the here and now. The following selection of symptoms illustrates Krypton's direct connection to the cosmic source, the centre of the universe around which all revolves. Note words in bold.

I felt I had an amazing touch of insight, clarity and creativity. I had a feeling of being able to **create**. It was as if there was no **separation** between creator and created; I feel in **sync** with the universe.

Dream I landed onto the highest place from somewhere in the universe to the **highest** mountain where I encountered glaciers of pure whiteness, and I was **descending** holding by the hand and talking to my daughter as two unpolluted loving souls. The landscape was very dramatic: full of beauty, danger and unity. A very clear sense of direction, experiencing that deep engorgement of happiness when being with a fresh soul of a child in such a journey, **descending** towards the lower plains of existence.

I connected with my father's journey; I saw him as if he had taken off as a rocket after his death. As if the **highest** self – spirit – has gone far beyond any human dimension, passed the sun and after this **ascent** with lots of light, he had **crashed** with some elements and come back to earth.

While compiling his system of the universe, he felt that he was following God's sequence of his thoughts, and the same impression of the existence of some **ultimate truth** grows inevitably.

I am everything that was and is and shall be, nor has any mortal ever uncovered my veil.

Feel serene inside.

Krypton has descending from above, an alien or a new soul on the peak of the highest mountain, in sync with God, the universe, the higher self and ultimate truth.

The spirituality of Krypton as brought out in the proving focuses on three different spiritual approaches. These are ancient Egyptian mythology and architecture, the biblical account of creation, and Tibetan Buddhism. I will examine each in relation to the proving, and look to the aspects that can enhance our understanding of Krypton's inner nature. My discussion is restricted to what I perceive to be significant to the understanding of Krypton. A deeper exposition of these doctrines is beyond the scope of this book and easily available on the internet or even from a guru.

Ancient Egypt

> *Be upright in thy whole life; be content in all its changes; so shalt thou make thy profit out of all occurrences; so shall everything that happeneth unto thee be the source of praise.*
>
> Akhenaton (King of Egypt, 14th century BC)

> *Know the world in yourself. Never look for yourself in the world, for this would be to project your illusion.*
>
> Luxor Temple Proverbs[3]

The Krypton proving presents several connections to ancient Egypt.

Repeated dreams of Karnak in Egypt.

Dreams of crypts and things being cryptic and coptic, of Egypt and Osiris.

Sensation of being in 14 parts, each disconnected from the others ... Osiris was an Egyptian, he was cut into 14 pieces, the torso is quartered.

Dream of losing my Egyptian Eye of Horus charm beside a stream.

Voices Karnak it's not the ark but the arc – arc lights, alignments carnac.

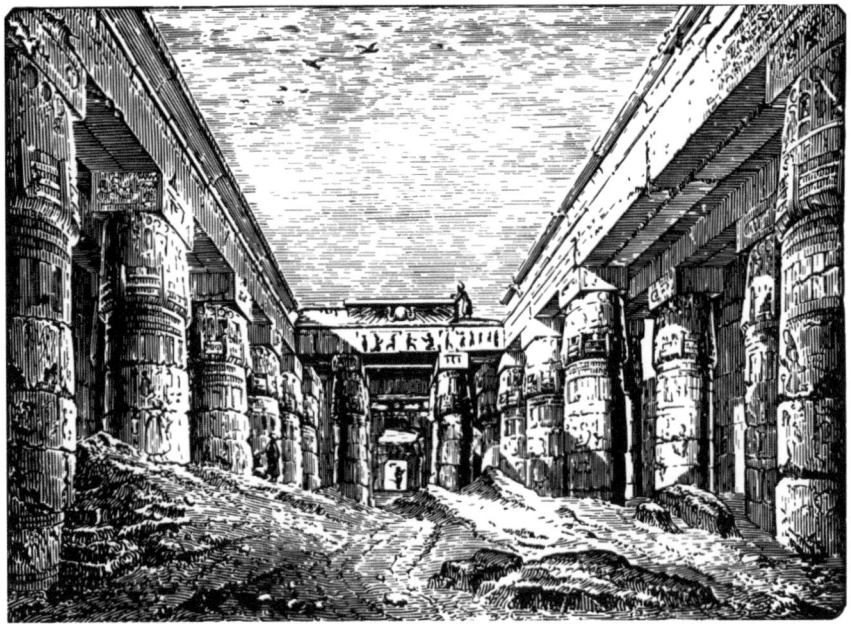

Figure 8.1 Karnak temple, Egypt

Ancient Egyptian concepts – Karnak[4]

First built to worship Montu, the god of war and the sky, in the 12th dynasty the large central site of Karnak, an ancient Egyptian temple compound was dedicated to Amun-Ra, the primeval one, the king of the deities and the God of Air and Sun. Surrounding his sanctuary were other areas devoted to his wife, Mut; to Montu, the falcon-headed god of war; Aten, the sun disk, and other deities.

As a model of the cosmos, and the meeting point of humans and gods, the temple was carefully aligned to the sun, moon, stars, and planets. Its main east/west axis may have enabled it to indicate both the midwinter sunset and sunrise in BCE 2000–1000, signifying the triumph of light over darkness. The temple was also oriented with the stars, especially Ursa Major, Vega and Arcturus, and the rituals included Ursa Major, Orion and the new moon. Sirius, the dog star, was used to predict the time of flooding of the Nile.

Because the stars move position, the Karnak temples were altered to keep up with the precise location of their aligned stars and to match the astronomical progression of the constellations. Montu, the bull, was replaced by the Amon ram coinciding with the age of Taurus moving into the age of Aries.

The geometric latitude of Karnak is 12.857°, deriving from the mathematical calculation 90° / 7.

Extraterrestrials

Karnak, the pyramids, and other ancient Egyptian structures are so meticulously detailed and so precisely oriented to the stars that some authors believe these extraordinary architectural feats could only be achieved with the help of aliens or extraterrestrial beings, who appeared as gods, instructing and influencing the locals. Erich von Däniken in his book *Chariots of the Gods*,[5] cites the world-wide phenomena of artwork depicting space vehicles, alien life-forms, and ancient astronauts. That this art was similar in far distant cultures around the world such as Stonehenge, Easter Island, Egypt, and Maya, adds to the belief that aliens were involved. In addition, several religious texts and traditions refer to aliens visiting from the stars and using space and air transport.

The Bible states:

> The Nephilim (giants) were on the earth in those days, when the sons of God went to the daughters of humans and had children by them.
>
> Genesis 6:4[6]

Naturally these theories have many critics and fall within the category of strange, rare and peculiar.

Osiris

Osiris was a powerful Egyptian god, who governed the afterlife, the underworld, the dead, resurrection, and vegetation. Linked with the constellation Orion and the star Sirius at the start of the new year, he ruled over the annual flooding and receding of the Nile and the regrowth of the crops.

He was the son of the Earth god and the Sky goddess, and simultaneously the brother and husband of Isis. One myth says that after he was killed by his brother, he was cut into 14 parts and spread throughout Egypt. Isis renewed his life by collecting and wrapping together the parts, confirming Osiris's association with resurrection and life. Isis then gave birth to their posthumously conceived son, Horus.

Horus and the Eye of Horus[7]

Horus, the son of Osiris and Isis, was the falcon-head Egyptian god of the sun and sky. He assisted his mother, Isis, in collecting and healing the severed parts of his father, Osiris, and then killed his uncle who had

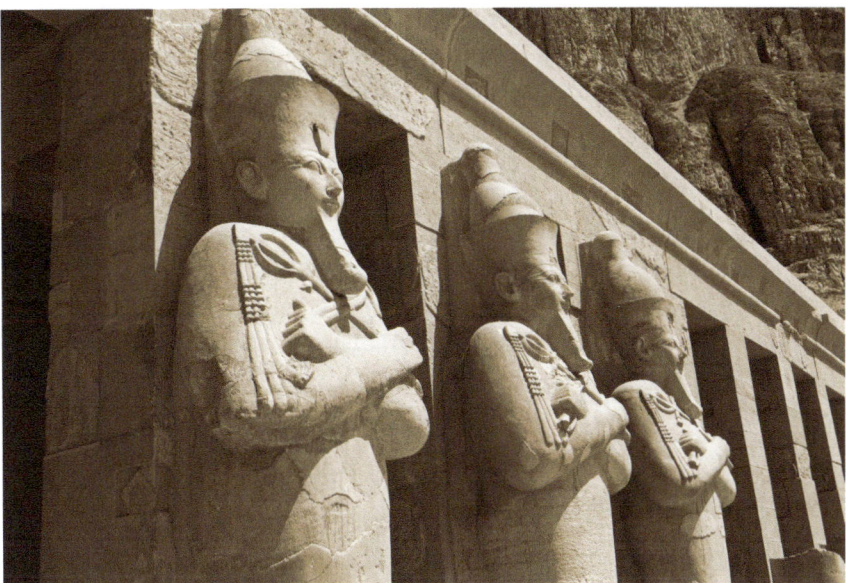

Figure 8.2 *Osiris*

murdered Osiris. In this battle Horus's left eye was damaged and then healed. Because of his brave actions, Horus was honored by the Egyptians with the **Eye of Horus**, a symbol of protection from evil and regeneration of health and wholeness. Egyptians created amulets and painted images of the Eye of Horus to ward off evil, such as on sea voyages, and to ensure good health and wellness.

The depiction of the Eye of Horus is composed of 6 parts,[8] measured in fractions with denominators of the powers of two: the right side of the eye = 1/2, the pupil = 1/4, the eyebrow = 1/8, the left side of the eye = 1/16, the curved tail = 1/32, the teardrop = 1/6 (Figure 8.3). Scholars have found that

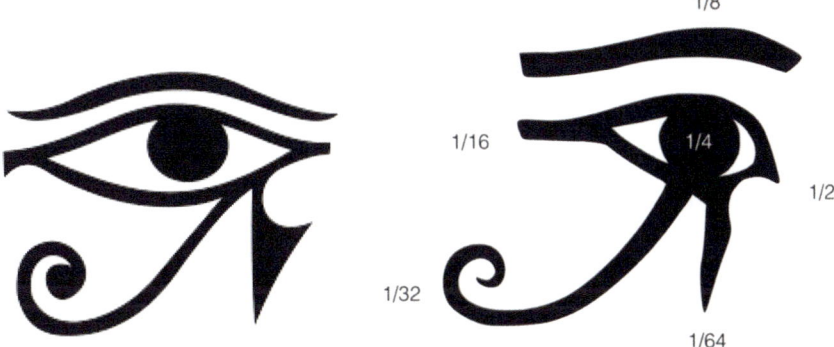

Figure 8.3 *The Eye of Horus*

the Eye symbol, when superimposed on an image of the mid-brain, is neurologically aligned with the areas of the six senses, the sixth sense being 'thinking', as the Eye of Horus was also known as the Eye of the Mind.

Carnac[9]

Located near the village of Carnac in France, is the ancient site of megalithic stone-circles and alignments, with over 3,000 stones. Carnac is situated on a unique latitude at which the solstice sun, both summer and winter, form a perfect Pythagorean triangle relative to the parallel of latitude, that is to the east–west axis of the site. The site is said to have originated 2,000 years before Pythagoras.

Cracking the hieroglyphic code

Finally, a reference to hieroglyphic code and the stars.

When we bought the material we thought the patterns were hieroglyphics ... but it turned out they were inverted star signs.

The Egyptian hieroglyphic code was one of the hardest of all to crack.[10] Early attempts by the 5th century scholar, Horapollo, to correlate the hieroglyphs with Egyptian allegories were inaccurate and misled scholars for centuries. British scholar, Thomas Young, made some progress in 1814, when he identified the marks indicating a pharaoh's name, but he gave up, not understanding the nature of the code.

It was the work of the French polylinguist, Jean-François Champollion, who in the early 1800s finally deciphered hieroglyphic inscriptions on the famous Rosetta Stone, that opened up the ancient language to the world and earned Champollion the title, "Father of Egyptology".

Champollion, a typical Krypton personality, was destined to reach this great achievement as a child prodigy in linguistics and a young student fascinated with Egyptian history, culture and hieroglyphics. At his birth a magician declared that Champollion would be famous and later he dedicated his life to this study, claiming he would be the first to translate the Egyptian script.

Examining the symbols on an old Egyptian cartouche, Champollion, deciphered the name of the pharaoh Ramses by comparing the characters to ancient Coptic, a written and spoken language, and confirmed his hypothesis that the pictorial symbols represented phonetic sounds, not the ideological or mystical meanings that earlier scholars had believed. He had cracked the code. 'Champollion was so overwhelmed by his discovery that he fainted on the spot.'

He then applied this knowledge to decoding the inscriptions on the Rosetta Stone, an ancient monument stone from 196BC discovered by the French that had a decree written in three different languages, including Egyptian hieroglyphs. By translation and cross-reference with the other two languages, Champollion cracked the code even further and provided the key to the modern understanding of Egyptian hieroglyphs.

Summary: ancient Egypt

The Krypton proving brings up several references to ancient Egyptian mythology, architecture, astronomy, and hieroglyphics. These relate well to the Krypton aspects regarding stars, time cycles, precise measurements, mathematics, and codes, not to mention extra-terrestrials. Egypt represents an extremely developed intellect in one of mankind's earliest civilisations. It was the dawn and blossoming of logic, yet with a strong connection to the heavens and the development of consciousness.

The following are a selection of quotes from the ancient Temple of Luxor:[11,12]

If you search for the laws of harmony, you will find knowledge.

Man, know yourself ... and you shalt know the god/dess.

Leave him in error who loves his error.

Know the world in yourself. Never look for yourself in the world, for this would be to project your illusion.

Knowledge is not necessarily wisdom.

The Bible

Wednesday

Walking
the cool African morning
my daily recurring ritual,
Sun rising red
threatening
to bake my day,
I turn the corner to find
a full moon in proud opposition,
holding its own
refusing to sink, or even pale.
Having chanced this monthly wonder
I stood, facing north Kilimanjaro snows.
Moon left, Sun right
cool pale, yellow warm
Fertilising my being
Entwining, coiling, rising.
One God.

Figure 8.4 Day Four of creation

In the previous volumes of this series, we examined the correspondences between the first three days of creation to Helium, Neon and Argon respectively. It follows that we should look for associations between the proving of Krypton, culminating the fourth period, and the fourth day of creation. Once again, the similarity is striking. What is important is not only to highlight these similarities but to extract the meaning that arises from them towards a deeper understanding of Krypton, its related fourth period, the Biblical story of creation and the nature of the world around us.

Let us start with the number four. Numbers are a big part of the Krypton proving, and four and its multiples are prominent.

Thoughts about the heart. Hearts are quartered like the 4 quarters of Jerusalem. Blake was talking about the fourfold division of Jerusalem – every part and thing and person is in 4 quarters.

Dream that Keppler explained to me his three laws, and what was the fourth?

The Fourth Day recounts the story of God's creation of the sun, moon and stars, all of which feature strongly in the proving of Krypton.

> And God said: 'Let there be lights in the firmament of the heaven to divide the day from the night; and let them be for signs, and for seasons, and for days and years; and let them be for lights in the firmament of the heaven to give light upon the earth.' And it was so. And God made the two great lights: the greater light to rule the day, and the lesser light to rule the night; and the stars. And God set them in the firmament of the heaven to give light upon the earth, and to rule over the day and over the night, and to divide the light from the darkness; and God saw that it was good.[13]

The sun, moon and stars are major aspects of both Krypton and its corresponding Fourth Day of Creation, which in itself is remarkable. More so is the relationship to time, which is also an important feature of the proving. The role of the heavenly bodies is not only to shine, but to mark time. It is by the sun, moon and stars that we measure the time and seasons.

Dream someone was juggling the 4 elements, someone is stringing the seasons together.

Time is not equal and there are still points for entering the Stargates.

A well-known conflict arises in the reading of the previous biblical passage, and it is a matter of sequence. The question regards the creation of light: '... *and let them be for lights in the firmament of the heaven to give light upon the earth*'.[14]

Hadn't God already created light in Day One? How come he is creating light again? There are several explanations. We may say that the first light was that of the Big Bang or the creation of photons shortly after, around 13.7 billion years ago. The sun and solar system appear around eight to nine billion years after the Big Bang, the difference representing the first four days on the biblical time scale. A parallel explanation by biblical interpreters is that the light of the first day was purely spiritual, while the light of the Fourth Day is material light. The light of the First Day came before the creation of the barrier between heaven and earth, the firmament, while the light of the Fourth Day emanates from the stars, which are themselves located within the firmament. However, how can we explain Day Three? How did the plants grow before there was light for photosynthesis? There had to be light, and it could not be entirely spiritual.

While the previous interpretations provide an interesting point of view, I find them to be somewhat lacking. I will present my own explanation.

A close examination of the Hebrew text shows the usual inadequacy of the English translation. The word *Maor* – 'lighting body' or 'luminary' is used, which is different from the word 'Or' used for light in the First Day. It is the difference between a light bulb and the light it emits. It is the bulb that was created on Day Four; light already existed. *'Let there be lights'* should read let there be light bodies, 'vessels' for concentrating and transferring the light.

The Hebrew meaning of 'Ma-or' may also be translated as 'What kind of light?'. It is a different aspect of light. So, while light was created on the First Day, the repositories or transmitters of light were only created on the Fourth Day. From an astrophysics point of view, this means photons came before stars, which is the correct sequence.

The more important aspect of the Fourth Day is timekeeping: *'to divide the day from the night; and let them be for signs, and for seasons, and for days and years'*.[13] The passage of time, day and night, sun and moon years, seasons and special events, are all measured by the heavenly bodies. Hence, the real creation of Day Four is the creation of time.

Did time not exist before? It did, but in a different configuration. The following is my humble interpretation:

Time can take many formats. When we measure it, we are looking for cycles of time, repetitive patterns that we can recognise and 'clock'. No cycle – no can measure. Day Four creates cycles. Patterns and cycles are a function of circular motion, i.e., rotation. Take light-years as an example. Light-years measure how far light travels in a year. But to measure a year we need cycles. The same goes for anything between a millisecond and an aeon. Once time re-cycles we can 'time' and quantify it. Hence, we may say that on Day Four measurement was created, which we have already seen is an important aspect of Krypton.

There was a conversation about 12 years between Keppler and Newton, and they were discussing the word "**scale**" and coming up with four meanings – **scale** was a balance, climb, proportion, and covering.

Scale is also an instrument of measurement. We measure 'Time zero' from GMT.

Dream of the Greenwich Naval College.

The cycles of days, nights, weeks, months, years, special events, and comets are all a function of rotational motion. It is this motion that was introduced in Day Four. Light already existed before, and if there was a before, so did time. But these forces were linear, and hence produced no perceivable pattern. Light could shine (Helium), time could flow in a line (Neon), seeds could grow (Argon); but they could not revolve or repeat. And this, my friends, is the hidden essence of Krypton. Repetition as opposed to linear motion, line bending into a circle.

As I curled up, I went through the ages of time.

I thought that if they see time as being curved then lines always come together anyway.

As opposed to the first day when I wanted to stretch out, I know wanted to curve like a fossil.

Slept curled up as a fossil shape and as a still as a fossil can be.

Dream I was doing the same thing repeatedly, time after time.

The overlap between Einstein and Keppler is to do with Carbon 12 and generations of stars. ... This is to liberate us from repetition.

But by what means does God create rotation? The cycles of the earth and its spin all depend on gravity. Without gravity, the planets would travel in straight lines and the earth would not spin. Nor would it tilt. We would lose the cycles of day and night, the seasons and the years.

From a cosmological perspective, gravitation causes dispersed matter to coalesce, and coalesced matter to remain intact, thus accounting for the existence of planets, stars, and galaxies.[15]

No gravity, no stars and planets.

Gravity is the force that curves spacetime and, consequently, light. If it were not for gravity, linear light would travel its straight and wearisome path for evermore. It was Einstein who realised that not only can light be bent, but so can time. This happens when space-time-light cruises too close to an intense gravitational force, such as a black hole. Hence, we can say that all God needed to do on the Fourth Day was to introduce gravity.

It felt like an irresistible force – the pull of gravity, but also connectedness.

There was a conversation between Keppler and Newton Einstein and a very irritable Rabbi. They talked about gravity for the rest of the night.

When gravity is created, things start to fall from the sky.

Dream of a falling star.

If a man falls off a plane in the middle of the night, only God can help him.

Einstein realised that the property of spacetime which is responsible for gravity is its *curvature*.[16] Space and time in Einstein's universe are no longer flatlands (as assumed by Neon-**Newton**) but can be pushed and pulled, stretched and warped by matter. Einstein didn't believe gravity was a force at all, but rather a distortion in the shape of space-time, otherwise known as "the fourth dimension". Gravity is strongest where spacetime is most curved, and it vanishes where spacetime is flat. The earth circles the sun because this is the shortest distance in curved three-dimensional spacetime. This is the core of Einstein's theory of general relativity, which is often summed up as follows: "Matter tells spacetime how to curve, and curved spacetime tells matter how to move".[15] Note that the curve introduced in the fourth day is not a curve of the first or second dimensions, i.e. line or surface. It is a curve of the third dimension, in other words warped volume, and as such belong to non-Euclidean geometry. Imagine a saddle, for instance. This topic will be further explored in Chapter 11 CM New dimensions. Hence, all God needed to create on the Fourth Day was a curve. The rest, including gravity, would follow.

Arc of light. Different qualities of light, scintillating light from fixed stars, curved light.

Spacetime-Light began to curve, curving closer and closer until it formed the tightly spun balls of light, the repositories of light. Hence, it is not the planets that create time, but curving and spinning spacetime that created the planets. For if they were not born of time, how could they mark its passage?

Dream fish were multiplying ... with one spinning so fast that it looked like 4.

We have established that Day Four-Krypton enables us to measure by creating cycles and patterns. Measuring requires intellect. It also breeds intellect. Measurement is the mother of logic. The first and foremost function of intellect is to measure, for without measure there can be no comparison, no similarity, no difference, no computations, and no considerations. In other words, the grand function of intellect is relativity.

So, we may say that on Day Four intellect was created. Or relativity.

It follows that if gravity – a cause and result of circular motion – was introduced on Day Four, and that if intellect was also introduced on Day Four, then intellect must be similar in quality to gravity. This would make intellect susceptible to curve, circular motion, and re-petition. Such an assumption may be brave or grave, a bonus with a heavy price. This is the price Krypton pays when it is locked in time grave spin.

Back to the biblical story. We see that the sun, moon and stars are located in the firmament, the same firmament that we met in Day Two and

Neon. Perhaps the real nature of the firmament is spacetime. There is a strong overlap between Neon and Krypton. But while Day Two presented a two-dimensional flat firmament, similar to the surface of water, Day Four curves the spacetime firmament.

Firmament spacetime is first and foremost a concept. Do not imagine it to be real, for its real is our imagination. There! The previous sentence is an example of curved thought. Enter the warp. We move from flatland Neon thought to curved Krypton intellect. Day Two gave birth to two-dimensional logic, the matrix. Day Four either curves logic into wisdom; or spins it into an intellectual loop, one that can measure, compare, or bore a hole into itself and others. God help us.

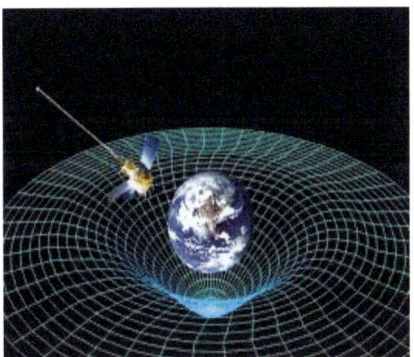 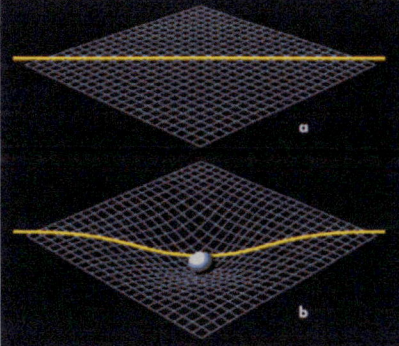

Figure 8.5 *Curved space time creating gravity*

There is another aspect to the Fourth Day. At the end of the narrative we find:

And God made the two great lights: the greater light to rule the day, and the lesser light to rule the night; and the stars. And God set them in the firmament of the heaven to give light upon the earth, and to rule over the day and over the night, and to divide the light from the darkness; and God saw that it was good.

Genesis 1:16[17]

For the first time we see a hierarchy appearing in the story of creation. God places the sun and moon to rule over the day and night. Actually, the Hebrew word is *memshelet* which means government. The sun and moon are not sole monarchs but part of a collective government. The sun and its collective forces govern the day; the moon and its collective forces govern the night and stars.

The word *memshelet* has another meaning. It is related to the word *mashal*, signifying metaphor or analogy. The sun and moon are analogous to the mind and emotions, respectively. The sun bears the light of truth, and the moon governs the flow of watery emotional tides in ebb and flow. The two are now separated: *To divide the light from the darkness.* We are governed by our conscious intellect by day and our emotions in the subconscious dark of night. From here on the two will do battle, as is apparent from the Krypton's predominance of either intellect or intuition. But the sun, the intellect, is the greater, a Krypton problem.

Both the sun and moon are our bodies' timekeepers; the pineal oscillates to the circadian beat, and the moon conducts the hormonal orchestra in its monthly rhythm.

Day Four

On the fourth day
God created the curve
And the curve brought forth
stars, moon, sun
spinning, cycling, marking time

So as to create these
heavenly bodies
all God needed
was to initiate gravity

When gravity was introduced
matter coalesced into planets
stars fused, galaxies swirled
black holes tempted red dwarfs.

To create gravity
all God needed
was to warp spacetime.

God leaned forward and
with one finger
imperceptibly
touched the firmament.

Spacetime curved
gravity pulled
light bent; time coiled
planets formed
intellects measured themselves.

God
created the multiverse
with the minimum dose

Tibetan Buddhism

While one side of Krypton is an intense intellect, the opposing side is freedom from mind and the belief systems it creates. Krypton spans the tension between mind and non-mind. As such it relates directly to Tibetan Buddhism and other Eastern philosophies.

I bought a calendar of Tibetan paintings.

I kept seeing mandalas.

Suddenly all systems of belief have disappeared, I have no belief anymore, it feels a big empty space now since the belief occupied so much! Everything belongs to this state of non-belief. A freeing view of beliefs. As everyone talks from belief, it becomes clear to discuss central matters to each person. The present infinite and no belief! Flowing, fluidity feeling of existence.

I heard the word *dzogchen*: the realisation of the nature of the mind. We were on the roof of the world to open the roof of the mind. The roof of the mind is open. No mind seeing the view, seeing with the third eye. True nature of thoughts as they rise, like waves, then sink back into the ocean and the gaps between thoughts.

Seeing things as they are, absolute state – knowing that the true nature of the mind is the true nature of everything.

Seeing absolute truth, the true nature of our mind. The five wisdoms cut through our conceptual mind. We create our own disease, our belief systems. We believe our mind is separate from the universal mind. The first separation is being aware of nakedness, that first split, the first delusion of duality, separating from the masculine and vice versa.

Love is the greatest expression of the divine – it is all encompassing. There are 12 senses.

The blind spot in the eye exists for the mind to see the truth.

A vision of Garuda,[i] born fully grown, just need to break the shell, not discard the body. The nature of the mind is deathless and eternally pure. To become more ordinary, not extraordinary. The extra creates a more elaborate, deluded vision, more intricate confusion. We are obsessed with theories, we miss the point. Why do we not recognise the nature of the mind? There are four reasons – we are too close, too profound, too easy, too amazing. A Seer is just seeing in. All the time we are looking outside ourselves. It's too close, the nose gets in the way.

---

[i] In Hindu mythology, the bird (a kite or an eagle) and the vahana (mount) of the god Vishnu. *Garuda*. Available online at: https://www.britannica.com/topic/Garuda

Waking dream of sitting alone on a vast plateau, and the Dalai Lama came to me grinning. He talked about a state of fresh virgin, unaltered by even a hair's breadth of concept. A luminous, naked awareness between thoughts. The word he used was *trekchš.* and he said it was cutting through delusion. Laying bare the primordial purity and natural simplicity of the nature of mind. The last word he said was *tšgal.*

Chanting in the evening Tibetan Buddhist mantras while driving. The sound that created broke my sound barrier.

PHAT! A word used to bring a corpse back to life. Also used backwards TAHP. It is not to be said aloud so you encode it.

I can easily imagine the following locations in the lofty Tibetan mountains.

Dream I landed onto the highest place from somewhere in the universe to the highest mountain where I encountered glaciers of pure whiteness.

Waking dream of sitting alone on a vast plateau, and the Dalai Lama came to me grinning.

Tibetan Buddhist concepts

Dzogchen[18]

In Tibetan Buddhism Dzogchen is the highest state of enlightenment, which has existed since the beginning of time and includes all the teachings and practices that are necessary to reach that state. It reflects the belief that all sentient beings in the universe contain the qualities of perfection, namely, indestructibility, purity, openness, clarity, simplicity, presence, and equality, that allow everyone to awaken to Great Perfection or Great Completeness. The analogy given by *Dzogchen* masters is that one's nature is like a **mirror** which reflects with complete openness, but is not affected by the reflections. The compassion and wisdom of the Buddha showed that he was already fully enlightened and fully aligned. These concepts of alignment, spirituality, and perfection of the master have a strong relationship to the noble gases in general and to Krypton in particular.

The Five Wisdoms[19]

The Five Wisdoms are aspects of the wisdom found in the state of Great Perfection.

1 The wisdom of all-encompassing space, the womb of compassion;
2 The mirror-like wisdom which has the capacity to reflect in precise detail whatever comes before it is;
3 The equalizing wisdom – the fundamental lack of any bias toward any impression;
4 The wisdom of discernment – the ability to distinguish clearly, without confusing the different phenomena that arise;
5 The all-accomplishing wisdom, which is the potential of having everything accomplished, perfected, and spontaneously present.

Garuda

In Tibetan Buddhism the Garuda is a mythical bird representing wisdom and the already existing state of perfection in all people. While the bird is fully developed in the egg and is born fully-grown, only when it hatches can it soar into the sky. In the same way, when the enlightened one discards his body like the bird sheds its shell, the fully-enlightened qualities are radiantly revealed.[20]

The Union of Skillful Means

There are two paths to Dzogchen, Kadak, purity of mind and Lhundrup, spontaneous presence from which all phenomena arise and return. Together they are referred to as the union of skillful means, a way of teaching about truth, and wisdom.[21]

PHAT

One of the practices of Dzogchen is the making the sound of PHAT, which disrupts thinking and attachments and brings the practitioner into a state of emptiness and clarity.[22]

Summary of Tibetan Buddhism

Three things cannot be long hidden: the sun, the moon, and the truth.

Buddha[23]

Previously we examined the computer-like intellect of Krypton. Precision measuring, code-cracking, star-gazing, computer-nerding, asper-berging – this intelligence can be a wonderful asset or a vicious cycle of disconnected heart and meaningless boredom. We saw two opposite sides of Krypton, one being the animal, leopard-skinned basic instinct, Freud's id. At the other end of this spectrum, we now find the superego, the highest spiritual nature of man, transcending beliefs and logical thought patterns while striving for the loftiest noble perfection. Its main spiritual focus is on the limitations of mind and the existential delusion of perceiving reality through its lens. When we see beyond the fragments of truth that hold us in their captivity, we can align with the real nature of truth, the universal mind. This concept fits well with Buddhist teachings.

Interestingly, it has recently been discovered that Tibetans have genes from Denisovan ancestors, an extinct branch of the Homo genus that were around hundreds of thousands of years before the cognitive revolution of 70,000 years ago.[24] While other humans have this gene too, it is present in Tibetans in a much higher degree and allows them to live at high altitudes without a consequent thickening of the blood which can result in pathology. Perhaps they retained something of the 'simple mind' that our ancestors had before becoming homo Krypton, allowing them to reach spiritual altitudes without a thickening of the intellectual barriers.

In practice we might find Krypton patients either immersed in the spiritual or imprisoned by the intellectual, or in a conflict between the two. Often the Krypton patient may use one to gain the other, as in using the intellect to attain spirituality.

Conclusion to 10M

We should take care not to make the intellect our god; it has, of course, powerful muscles, but no personality.

Albert Einstein[25]

I have examined three different spiritual approaches as manifested in the Krypton proving: Egyptian astrological architecture, the biblical story of creation and Tibetan Buddhism. These deal with our relationship to cycles of time, stars, mind, and non-mind.

Egyptian architecture lines and aligns its logic with the stars. The Bible tells the story of the stars' creation, the conversion of space time from linear to cyclical. Tibetan Buddhism seeks to end striving by transcending logical cycles of Karma and belief. The progression is from line to curve to circle, and to the breaking of the cycle.

Ultimately all three explore the development of consciousness. The common denominator is time, straight, curved or circular, and the cycles of our intellect, that which can measure, build, and create belief systems to enhance or confine us. Our intellect can move in Neon flatland logic, or Krypton recycled mush, or the combination of both: curved spiraling wisdom.

In the next chapter we will further examine the intellect's nature.

References

1 Norbu CN. *Dzogche Quotes*. In: *Dzogchen: The Self-Perfected State*. Show Lion, 1996. Available online at: http://tinyurl.com/498nsf7z (accessed July 18, 2023).

2 Einstein A. *Brainy Quote*. Available online at: http://tinyurl.com/4zypbhnx (accessed July 18, 2023).

3 Akhenaton. *Golden Proverbs: Akhenaton Quotes*. Available online at: http://tinyurl.com/4nxz8tx8h (accessed July 18, 2023).

4 J Mark. Karnak. In: *World History Encyclopedia*. World History Publishing, 2016. Available online at: http://tinyurl.com/2zaea26e (accessed July 17, 2023).

5 Chariots of the Gods. *Wikipedia*. Available online at: http://tinyurl.com/mtk8f-s2f (accessed July 17, 2023).

6 Genesis 6:1–4. *Biblia*. Available online at: https://biblia.com/bible/esv/genesis/6/1-4 (accessed July 17, 2023).

7 Rose C. The Story of Osiris. Isis and Horus: The Egyptian Myth of Creation. *Academia*. Available online at: http://tinyurl.com/w7zyb3ma (accessed July 17, 2023).

8 ReFaey K, Quinones GC, Clifton W *et al*. The Eye of Horus: The Connection Between Art, Medicine, and Mythology in Ancient Egypt. *Pub Med Cureus*. May 2019. Available online at http://tinyurl.com/e9zc46xf (accessed January 22, 2024).

9 Whitaker A. The Carnac Complex. *Ancient Wisdom*. Available online at: http://tinyurl.com/ec3zh7uy (accessed July 17, 2023).

10 HowStuffWorks Contributors. What is the Rosetta Stone and Why is the Artifact Important? *Howstuffworks*. 15 September, 2023. Available online at: http://tinyurl.com/23ua6eav (accessed July 17, 2023).

11 Anon. Proverbs from the Luxor Temple of Amun Mut Mont. *Malaika Mutere*. Available online at: http://tinyurl.com/23j6e7z8 (accessed July 17, 2023).

12 Anon. Ancient Man: The Beginning of Civilizations. *Poetry for Every Occasion*. Available online at: http://tinyurl.com/mrxmst2d (accessed July 17, 2023).

13 Genesis 1:14. *Bible Hub*. Available online at: http://tinyurl.com/yeykt9cp (accessed July 17, 2023).

14   Genesis 1:15. *Brainly*. Available online at: https://brainly.com/question/ 18417272 (accessed July 17, 2023).

15   Gravitation. *Gravity Wiki*. Available online at: http://tinyurl.com/5cj73mpv (accessed July 17, 2023).

16   Einstein's Spacetime. *Gravity Probe B*. Available online at: http://tinyurl.com/ 38dzzhnf (accessed July 17, 2023).

17   Genesis 1:16. *Bible Hub*. Available online at: https://biblehub.com/genesis/1. htm (accessed July 17, 2023).

18   Dzogchen. *Wikipedia*. Available online at: http://en.wikipedia.org/wiki/Dzogchen

19   Sogyal Rinpoche. *The Tibetan Book of Living and Dying*, HarperOne, 200, p157.

20   Garuda. *Wikipedia*. Available online at: http://en.wikipedia.org/wiki/Garuda (accessed July 17, 2023).

21   Union of Skillful Means and Wisdom. Rigpa Shedra. Available online at: http:// tinyurl.com/bdh5bd6x (accessed July 17, 2023).

22   Reynolds J. *The Golden Letters: The Tibetan Teachings of Garab Dorje*. Ithica NY: Snow Lion Publications, 1996, p92.

23   The Socratic Method – *Buddha*. Available online at: http://tinyurl.com/ycxk2pya (accessed January 15, 2024).

24   Life at the top. *The Economist*, July 5, 2014. Available online at: http://tinyurl. com/mr3pzprb (accessed July 18, 2023).

25   Einstein A. *Brainy Quote*. Available online at: http://tinyurl.com/mr3pzprb (accessed July 18, 2023).

9

KRYPTON MEDITATION PROVING

The real danger is not that computers will begin to think like men, but that men will begin to think like computers.

Sydney J Harris[1]

I am a brain, Watson. The rest of me is a mere appendix.

Arthur Conan Doyle[2]

The following is a meditation proving done by my wife, Camilla, meaning she held but did not take the remedy. *She had no idea what the remedy was.* I find her provings to be extremely accurate, and they often shed light on deeper aspects of the remedy. The proving was recorded verbatim from the moment it began. Bold type words are my emphasis.

I feel cross want to frown. [She is frowning. JS]

I feel concentration between eyes, below the third eye.

My head feels like nothing is moving inside, thick, as if nothing in there. Numb in head, all in third eye [She is pressing hand to forehead, between and just above the eyes. From here on 'The third eye' refers to this point. JS]

No **Synapses**. Everything concentrated in front.

I feel like the Rodin statue, 'The Thinker'.

As if everything is too much and you can't think any more. As if everything is concentrated in the third eye and the rest of my head is vacant, a mass of brain with no connections. All the connections are in the third eye, a pain in the butt!

[Observation: Hand rubbing between eyes all the time.]

I feel like the ultimate European – all connections in the front lobe and frowning all the time, opposite of African people. Like someone who thinks a lot, and can only use this part of the brain, everything is logic: 'If A is this and B is that then C will happen.'

No higher knowledge or no connection to any other knowledge. Front brain people who massage this area and hold it a lot. Like a kind of a brain fag.

I am frowning between the eyes, frowning like a thinking frown.

[Massaging between eyes. Irritability. JS]

This is young knowledge. Not wisdom, just knowledge.

This person can't think, because he is thinking too much with this area, so the opposite happens. I feel completely out of it, just need to lie down, can't keep my eyes open. You have worked your brain so much that you need to sleep. Too much activity in the front of head, can't get over this part, it is so overwhelmingly prominent.

Feels like I am going cross-eyed.

Lots of neurological synapses in between eyes and nothing in the rest of head, the rest is not wired. This is like the ultimate human – the part of thinking and planning and logic, but we lost the rest of the knowledge of the whole brain, the old knowledge, the wisdom. The old part of the brain is not activated – you can't survive in the jungle, you don't trust your intuition. It's all just A-B-C-D, linear. All hyper-focused into the front, into the future, planning the future and thinking that it's important. Progress, progress and more progress for the sake of it, but you lose your connection to the past. Operating from a very small place and base, you cut all the connections to history, not learning from the past, but thinking you can only learn from the future, and really believing that this is progress, even though it is not. Everything is new.

My eyes are heavy and I have to close them.

If you were to light up my brain only this part would light up (the front between the eyes), where we frown.

This feels like someone for whom everything is new. You are not learning or functioning from prior knowledge, just using new knowledge and books and research. This makes my eyes very heavy.

It is as if the ancestors are cut off. All is new. No value to anything that is old or ancestral or prior knowledge, only now and the future. All the thought processes seem complex, but they are not conducive, not real but new limited knowledge, 'what happens if I do this or do that'. Like intelligence without wisdom. Someone thinking too much, exhausted, thinking as an exercise. Just action and reaction, action and reaction.

Photophobia. squinting against the light. Too much light coming in from here (front). the synapses there are burning so bright.

I am falling asleep and dreaming at the same time, but can't catch it.

Image of a lot of people coming towards me, kids running.

Someone who over-thinks, but it is primitive thinking, one way of thinking and not combining many ways of thinking, like a modern scientist, no wisdom, not learning from incarnations or ancestors, a new soul just using certain knowledge bases from the frontal lobe. Just experimental: 'If I kick the elephant in the ass what will it do?'. It is primitive but they think they are forward and forward thinking. But it is linear and doesn't take into account the whole brain, the old wisdom not activated. The ancient being doesn't get acknowledged at all; what other incarnations have taught us or what our ancestors have learnt. No regard for the old, just about new – very childish. But they think it's smart. They are smart, but very one-sided, not rounded. Linear, future-oriented. Idolising the future, idolising man, thinking man is so amazing.

They are dwarfed. simplistic, linear, future-oriented, all that is called scientific, idolising the new man, man's powers, but no wisdom. Like not giving chimps any credit.

Emotionally there is anxiety and anger. But this is not a very emotional being, more a rational being. A lot of abstract thinking but without prior knowledge, relying on your brain, but only part of your brain, and thinking that is the superior part.

Images of a woman I know, a top academic scholar, but frowning all the time, suppresses the intuitive part and not giving it much credit. She is a chimp and animal expert. Chimp and elephant, these are the two animals that came to me in this proving. We think we are so superior to animals, just because we use this part of the brain, everyone concentrating on it, like that it is the beginning and end of all, and neglects everything else. We don't trust them, or their intuition and knowledge. Just use your brain, frown, work hard at school – all wrong, but that is what makes us human these days. But Africans don't have that, they use the brain more holistically in a different way, but some people think it is inferior.

It may be that Asperger kids whose use of synapses are much wider in the brain but can't use this front part.

This remedy is knowledge but no feeling, disconnecting from it, just rational, like you marry someone because it makes sense. Very tired from using the brain too much!

After the proving

I feel light and happy, thank God I wasn't born like that! What a fucked up life, poor people! it was awful!

Note: After the proving, she gave the friend she mentioned a dose of Krypton, which worked very well. See Case 13.7 *Spiritual Scientist* (p 131).

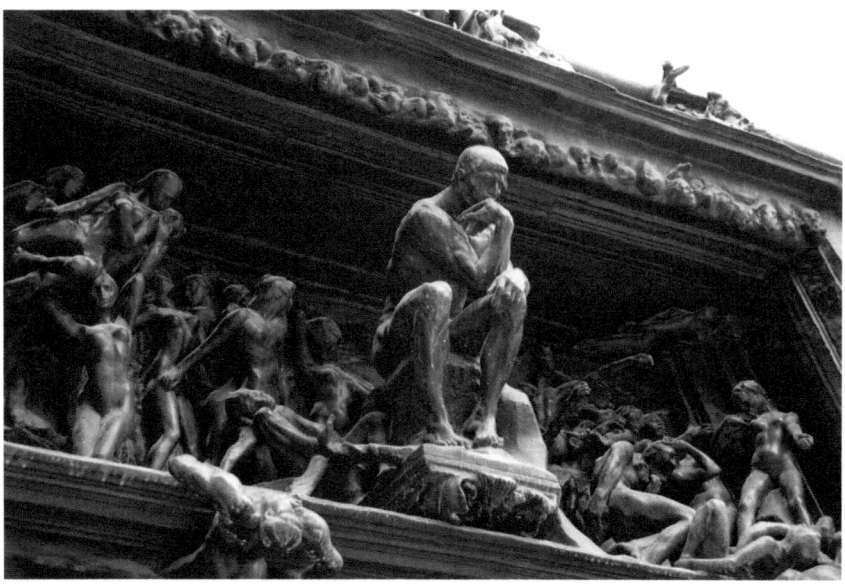

Figure 9.1 *The thinker at the gates of hell by Rodin*

Comment

> *Time moves in one direction, memory in another.*
>
> William Gibson[3]
>
> *I'd rather have a bottle in front of me, than a frontal lobotomy.*
>
> Dorothy Parker[4]

Once again, I was surprised and impressed with my wife's proving. I already knew that this remedy was highly intellectual at the expense of emotions, but the new information highlighted and explained various aspects.

From this proving, I further realised the connection between the direction of time flow and the intellect. While the time flow of ancient or intuitive knowledge is circular and holistic, under the influence of Krypton time flows in a linear direction towards the future. We might suppose that it flows from back forwards, towards the frontal lobe, but it is equally possible to say that on the contrary, time is relentlessly moving towards our face as we push forward into it. This depends on our point of view in relation to time, as it is all relative.

The Aymara were members of a great but little-known culture of the Americas centred in the ancient city of Tiahuanaco.[5] In contrast to most civilizations, to the Aymara the past appears before us and the future lies behind us. They claim that one can see the past, therefore it must be situated in front of our eyes, whereas the unknown future is hidden in the shadows behind us. They face the past with their backs to the future, so time flows backwards through them. Like many other aboriginal tribes, they live in 'dream time'.

In terms of being apsoric, the Aymara are also interesting as they are totally free from prejudice. They only believe in what they see. Thus, despite repeated attempts, missionaries were not able to convert the Aymara to Christianity, because they could not see Christ in person. As a people for whom time flows backwards, their logic also flows in an opposite direction to our conventions, and they refuse to see the 'invisible'.

It seems that at the evolutionary point of Krypton, the direction of time reverses, so that we put future in front of us, look forward to the future and believe our own brain to be supreme. This accords with the reversal and mirror writing of Krypton. As in the Tibetan aspects mentioned earlier, we attempt to 'cross our eyes'.

Following the proving with Camilla, I was heavily influenced and thoughts of Krypton continuously revolved in my brain. That night I had a dream in which I was holding two exposed wires with a high voltage electric current flowing through them. I could get a shock, but the question was, which direction was the current flowing? One direction shock, the other direction safe.

Once we pass through the mirror and the direction of time reverses, we are pushed to focus on the frontal lobe of our brain. The frontal lobe is associated with reasoning, motor skills, higher level cognition, emotional regulation, and expressive language. It also controls the executive functions, judgement and decision-making skills, motivation, and planning for the future. It governs the ability to choose between good and bad actions (or better and best), and to determine similarities and differences between things or events. In other words, cause, effect, comparison, and **measurement**. In humans, the frontal lobe contains areas unique to our species, such as complex language processing.

The brain develops in a back to front pattern, from simple to complex, both historically and in individuals. The frontal lobe reaches full maturity around the age of 25, resulting in the cognitive maturity associated with adulthood.[6] The frontal lobe decreases in volume with age. Recent research has raised the possibility that Neanderthals developed a smaller frontal lobe due to more area associated with visual processing because they had larger eyes.[7] These were necessary for vision in the dark European winters, as opposed to Homo sapiens, who evolved in light-flooded Africa with less brain space required for visual processing and more room to develop large frontal lobes.

We may recall that Argon left us at the point of maturation, around the age of 18. Krypton evolves us into the next stage, where planning, responsibility and work-related functions predominate, the age where the emotions of youth blossom into the intellect of maturity. The circular and wholesome magical world of childhood is now replaced by the linear adult world, the age of cognition. And it is marching grimly forward.

In historical terms, humanity evolved into this age about 70,000 years ago, demonstrating modern cognition and behavior.[8] That was when we departed from our place as equals among animals and started moving forward towards the supremacy of Homo sapiens – the wise man. In the light of recent human history, it is questionable whether 'wise' is the right adjective. Perhaps the 'stuck in a thinking loop man' would be appropriate. In Swahili, the word for the white man is *Mzungu*, literally 'those with vertigo' or 'those who walk around in circles'. This circular thinking is the cradle of chronic disease, the cerebral trap we have locked ourselves into.

As I curled up I went through the ages of time.

Here we see a peculiar opposition. While it seems that in Krypton time and thought have become linear, the opposite side of going round in circles is also apparent. There are several ways to explain this contradiction. It may be that the thinking only appears to be linear, a delusion, while in fact it is going round in circles. Hence the many scientists who believe they are marching forward while in reality they are stuck in a loop. An example would be research I read proving that breast feeding is good for babies. Duh.

Another possibility might be that the circular time of Krypton has become confined to the frontal lobe, splitting into two extremes: repetitive circular thinking side by side with linear 'logical' thought. While before Krypton the mind was a gently curving harmonious sinus wave, it has now separated into line and circle.

If all this seems like an impossible Escher-like logical conundrum, that is exactly the nature of Krypton patients and the type of thought they delight in churning.

The comparison of old human thought patterns to animal thought is apparent in the proving, and echoes the animal theme of the remedy, such as a desire to wear leopard skin clothes. The images of elephant and chimp in this meditation proving represent the wisest and smartest of animal power.

In *The Dynamic Materia Medica of the Noble Gases: Argon*,[9] I concluded that the power of the Tree of Knowledge resulted from its ability to reverse the direction of time's flow. Before eating from this tree, Adam and Eve would live forever; hence, the Tree of Life was not forbidden. Eating from

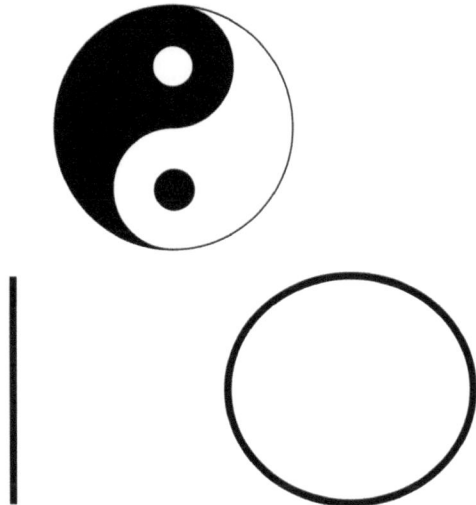

Figure 9.2 *Harmony separating into line and circle*

it would have no impact on them. Only the Tree of Knowledge was forbidden, as eating from its fruit meant ultimate death, the disease of 'Chronos' or time. The point of eating the fruit of knowledge is analogous to Krypton, when our eyes open to illuminate our frontal lobe, and we revolve to face our other half (see *Helium*, the point of cross over). Enter the mirror. This mirror is our shadow side, the shadow which Argon's Peter Pan can still lose but becomes permanently attached to us as we grow older.

Krypton, the fourth noble gas, has three noble elements above and three below, hence it is the fulcrum, the point of cross over from ancient to modern, from childhood to maturity, from innocence to sexuality, from life-wards to deathwards, from acute to chronic, from playground to mortgage. It is the point of stepping through the mirror, where the world crosses over and becomes cryptic.

From town to city

I awoke thinking "Where is Mesopotamia"?

Previously, I mentioned the emerging of higher cognition as a parallel to the Krypton stage in mankind's history. Until this stage, we were living as one particular species among the animals, and not a very successful one. Although they had the use of tools and fire, humans were simple gatherers of little distinction, and were hunted by many predators. They lived as underdogs, in constant fear. A chimp could easily kill a human, more so a lion or tiger.

Around 100,000 years ago there were several human species, such as *Homo erectus, Homo floresiensis, Homo ergaster, Homo denisova,* and *Homo neanderthalensis. Neanderthals* in many ways were more successful models than our species, *Homo sapiens.* Pound for pound a Neanderthal could rip a Sapiens apart, had a brain just as big, used tools and fire and could withstand cold climates better.[10] In fact, the Neanderthals had successfully vanquished the Sapiens in the Middle East some 100,000 years ago. One-zero to the Neanderthals. Yet Homo sapiens eventually eradicated the Neanderthals, and subdued all other human species and animals to become the supreme ruler of the planet. How did this happen?

Until 70,000 years ago, the maximum number of people that could cooperate effectively, known as Dunbar's number, was around 150. According to Pathmuditha, this is the *number of people you would not feel embarrassed about joining uninvited for a drink if you happened to bump into them in a bar.*[11] More than that would result in confusion and faction fighting. This is still true for animals. When the group grows too large, its social order destabilises and splits. The number is even smaller for larger mammals. It is rare for a chimpanzee group to number more than one hundred members. Ants and bees can cooperate in large numbers, but they do so in a very fixed manner. How did Homo sapiens manage to cross this critical threshold, and eventually set up cities comprising tens of thousands of inhabitants, and empires with hundreds of millions of people? There are several theories.[12] One is that with human brain size, cognitive ability and intelligence increasing over generations, they gained skills in living in larger groups from cultural information exchange and social learning.

References

1   Harris SJ. *Sydney J Harris Quotes.* Available online at: http://tinyurl.com/3c5p-kbh5 (accessed July 18, 2023).
2   Doyle AC. In: The Adventure of the Mazarin Stone. *Strand Magazine,* 1921. Quote available online at: http://tinyurl.com/4h78rufx (accessed July 18, 2023).
3   Gibson W. In: *Distrust that particular Flavor* (2012). Quote available online at: http://tinyurl.com/4untsrc4 (accessed July 18, 2023).
4   Parker D. *Dorothy Parker Quotes.* Available online at: http://tinyurl.com/48dsyfd2 (accessed July 18, 2023).
5   Aymara. *Encyclopedia.com.* Available online at: http://tinyurl.com/mvhyh2ve (accessed 24 January, 2024).
6   Haque M., Arian M, Johal N *et al.* Maturation of the Adolescent Brain. *Neuro-psychiatric Disease Treatment,* 2013, 9: 449–481. Abstract available online at *Pub Med:* http://tinyurl.com/bdz2p7we (accessed July 17, 2023).
7   Ghosh P. Neanderthals Large Eyes Caused Their Demise. *BBC News.* 13 March, 2013. Available online at: http://tinyurl.com/ymjxt4ar (accessed July 17, 2023).

8   Wayman E. When did the human mind evolve to what it is today? *Smithsonian Magazine*, June 25, 2012. Available online at http://tinyurl.com/5ffdhk63 (accessed July 18, 2023).

9   Sherr J. *The Dynamic Materia Medica of the Noble Gases: Argon*. Glasgow: Saltire Books, 2018.

10 Blaxland B. The First Migrations Out of Africa. *Australian Museum*, April 3, 2020. Available online at: http://tinyurl.com/r8pz4p36 (accessed July 18, 2023).

11 Pathmuditha I. Dunbar's Number. *Medium*, April 2, 2019. Available online at: http://tinyurl.com/2atpn7jx (accessed July 18, 2023).

12 Leytham-Powell C. Survival of the Socially Fittest. *Sapiens*, February 1, 2016, Available online at: http://tinyurl.com/2cs2mwyv (accessed July 18, 2023).

10

KRYPTON 50M: SENSATION, FUNCTION, STRUCTURE, GEOMETRY

We now leave the realm of affinities and emotions, nouns and adjectives, spirit and intellect, and move to the realm of verbs, which deal with the position, geometry and movement of bodies in time and space. Our sensations, mediated by the nervous system, sense our position in time-space. Verbs or functions are the response with a counter-motion of the vital force.

The geometry of Krypton neatly echoes the themes of its noble parent, grandparent, and great grandparent: Argon, Neon, and Helium. This may be synthesised as:

Being aligned with the vertical axis

This vertical axis is the line that connects mid-heaven to center earth, the line of truth, here and now. If we are aligned with this axis, it should pass through our vertex, spine and perineum. From this position we revolve life rather than life revolving us. Imagine an old record player. You can sit on the still axis in the center, or you can be whizzed around the periphery and occasionally be thrown off the edge by life's centrifugal forces. This is the principle of Tai chi: stay centered upright and vertical, revolving around a central axis, and you become invincible.

Once aligned, we are spiritually connected with our mission on earth (Helium), full of bliss and vital energy (Neon), and flowing the unobstructed path of life and love (Argon). The sun is at noon position, and we view the world from directly above. There is no shadow side, just light. We stand tall, and powered by unlimited cosmic energy, everything is possible, and all happens in the right way, time, and place. Like a noble gas pumped with electricity, we literally light up. Welcome to the wonderful world of spiritual, mental, emotional, and physical upright nobility.

The following are some reminders, edited and arranged into *As If One Person*:

Helium

I feel very tall, as though I am towering over everything. I see myself in a very direct way, as if from the outside. I feel superior. I feel as though I have eyes all over my head, that I am all-seeing. I see very clearly, how things really are. I could change anything in the whole world by aligning myself with that love and bringing it into every situation in my life. I felt very purposeful. I am going through the process of following my heart and working from the will of God; It is all to do with work, direction, life purpose and what you achieve as an individual. My mission is the main thing in my life, I only want to do important things, no unnecessary conversation. Much less bad conscience about what I do and what people think about me. I see more clearly what my responsibility is. I have achieved all my dreams and desires and do not have anything else to strive for at present. I now feel very good, free to make my own choices. This is about giving birth to self and truth. I woke feeling universally loved, universal consciousness.

Neon

The whole proving can be described as a rectification. I now feel very upright in space; before I was at a slight tilt – both physically and morally. I feel so different in my body. A weight has been lifted; the bowed feeling has been replaced by uprightness. I was amazed at how huge I was. I was cruising along on an energy which was not of my own muscular power, it seemed as if it was coming from somewhere else. Walking was effortless, light and free, with a sensation of walking uniformly. Life felt blissful, no resistance, a harmony between heaven and earth, effortless. My mind is free of distractions and I feel contented, not wanting anything, totally un-needy. No difference between the observer and the observed. Everything seems more beautiful. Moments of universal happiness. I am all in the now. A sense of absolute oneness.

Argon

Pillars are mutually supportive when they're vertical. The truth is straight, deceit is crooked. Felt like things were up righting. I feel taller, in complete alignment, settled in the middle of my soul, body and emotions. The sun was always shining, granting power to be and to act. If the sun is directly above, there's no shadow. I feel above it all, looking down on the wonderful world. I could fly, like being carried by wings. Unbelievable smooth easiness. The feeling of things being in the right order, fit me back into place. Whatever you are is right for you. Totally directed in actions. A clear path ahead; a straight line. Very focused and methodical, achieving things that didn't seem achievable. Clarity of thought and deep connection. Energy high and focused. Feeling of flowing, going with the flow. Adapting to everything much more softly. A great sense of energy, power behind me, complete tasks, and objectives. A sense of freedom; of being allowed to do what I wish, with a clear straight river ahead.

Please do not rush off to take all the noble remedies at once. They will only be effective in the right time and place, remember there is another side to this nobility.

Back to Krypton. The following symptoms are accounts from different provers that show a remarkable consistency, not only in relation to the whole Krypton proving, but in relation to all of the noble gas provings (Xenon and Radon included).

We begin with the upright alignment of Krypton. As in the preceding nobles, Krypton stands tall, aligned with the vertical axis of life and truth, the central world axis.

Dream: – I landed onto the highest place from somewhere in the universe to the highest mountain.

I see a picture of a bald man with a horn growing on his vertex.

The roof of the mind is open. No mind seeing the view, seeing with the third eye.

On waking I had a desire to cut the centre of my hair on the crown, so that it was sticking straight up, so that I could transmit as well as receive.

Before falling asleep I moved to align myself directly with the stars through the sky window in my room. I joined the stars as I fell asleep.

MC – mid-heaven, master of ceremonies, masterclass.

Voices of Karnak, it's not the ark but the arc – arc lights, alignments Carnac. At midday, the light comes from the front of the house to the back – alignment.

Vertigo – this has been happening on and off – it is almost like a shift on the vertical hold – I can stop it by focusing firmly.

Figure 10.1 demonstrates the vertically aligned nobles as compared to the tilt of common elements. I have used the third period as an example since it is shorter and easier to understand (and draw). This idea is discussed more fully in the *Neon* and *Argon* books.

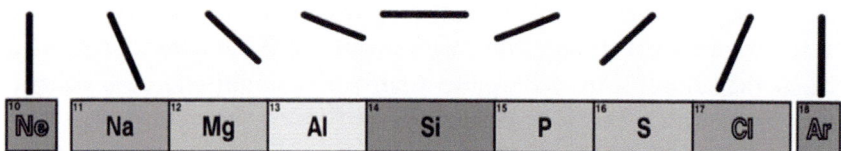

Figure 10.1 Vertical alignment of the noble elements, as opposed to the tilt of common elements

Elongation

With this alignment along the central vertical axis comes a sense of elongation. At this point Krypton is still similar to the first three nobles. That will change.

Sensation of feeling taller from crown of head upwards.

Images of very tall, elongated figures on going to sleep, similar to Giacometti sculptures.

I see a young exotic woman; her mandible is elongated.

Vision of a man's face, his nose is elongating rapidly, in a spiral-like motion upwards.

Top lip seems elongated, want to put tongue out and lick it like a lizard.

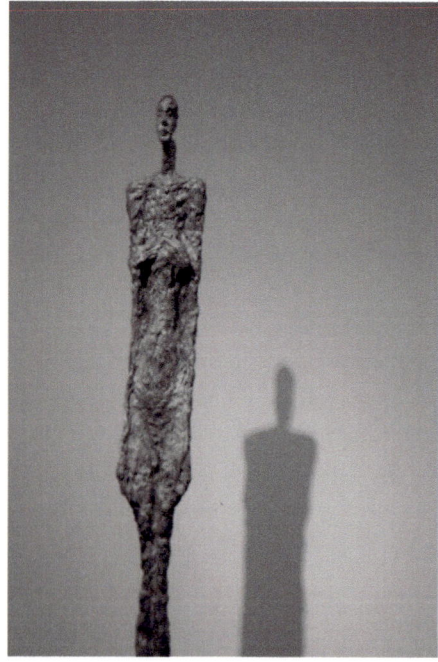

Figure 10.2 Giacometti woman of Venice II

Note that the elongation of Krypton is not only vertical. The chin and tongue are elongated horizontally, and the nose is also affected. Horizontal and vertical. This horizontal aspect also appears in the previous nobles, a negative opposition to the vertical line, with spiritual, mental and physical consequences. The Helium line may align horizontally, accompanied with prostration, apathy and inertia. In Neon a tilt results in being off center, living in the future or past and being controlled by desire and aversions. In Argon the horizontal axis leads to an obstruction of life's flow.

Curl – straight

An enormous force bends all lines into circles.

Joseph Chilton Pearce[1]

In the noble pathology the line cannot only prostrate itself, but it may also curl. We previously met this in Helium, and it reoccurs in Krypton. As in day four of creation, our straight line begins to curl.

The need to stretch my full body is back again.

Intensive need to curl up completely. I felt like the shape of a fossil.

As I curled up and I went through the ages of time.

A spiral staircase of a 3-floor building is moving in a drill-like motion beneath the ground.

Feel as if carrying a heavy weight on my back, like a person on my back. Uncomfortable to straighten up and stand tall, pressure on back is pushing me down. Feels as if I should walk bent over, so the weight would be on top of my back, but then my head feels awful, heavy, and muddled when leaning forwards.

As if the back just got turned three times around.

Severe low back pain, having to bend double to stand or walk.

I suddenly had pain in my back. Sensation as if two discs there had just slipped in opposite directions sideways; as if the spine had just separated at that point, and the upper and lower portions had moved in different directions sideways.

In pathology, the nobles tilt and curl. They become commoners, like the low-class elements. As we bend away from the universal vertical alignment, we veer from bowed to inert lying down. Whichever the case, not good. From the lofty vertical spiritual heights of the Tibetan mountains, we begin the slow and painful decent into a flat reality. Going down.

Sliding

I feel I'm sinking.

I feel I'm sliding down into somewhere, yet I have a feeling of tranquility – as if I don't give a damn about anything.

No energy, sliding down. The increase of sexual desire has gone. I've no energy. I feel I'm sliding into somewhere.

"Slip sliding away, Slip sliding away, the nearer destination the more you slip sliding away." The Concert in Central Park The song for the proving.

I recall a line from a poem by a well-known poet:

If a man falls off a plane in the middle of the night, only God can help him.[1]

This helpless sliding is the hallmark of chronic disease. You know where you were, you remember what was possible. But the gravity of life causes tilting and sinking and we can only offer helpless acceptance, there is nothing we can do. This is the sensation of Krypton as it disconnects from the one.

The horizontal aspect appears in Krypton in the form of 90 degrees, the right angle between noble vertical alignment and inert flat on back.

Right Angles

Dream of right-angles.

Celestial equators 90 degrees.

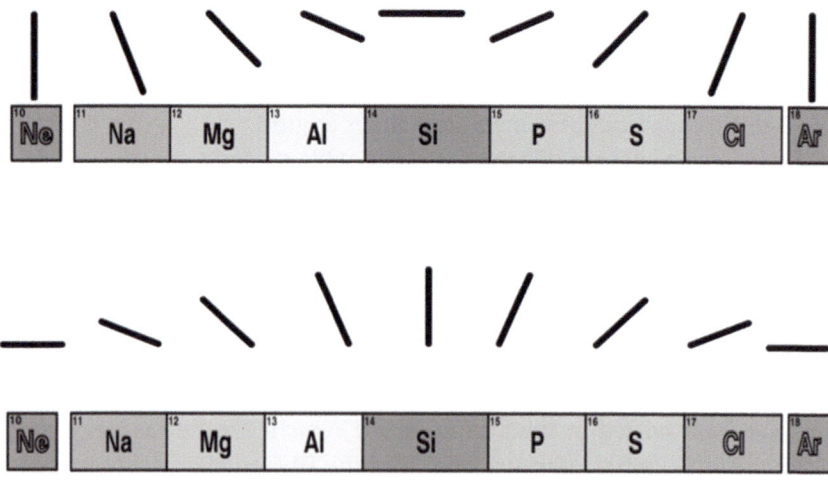

Figure 10.3 *Angles of the periodic table. From Noble vertical alignment to inert flat on back*

<hr />

[1] Quote is from a poem by the Israeli poet, translator, and peace activist, Dahlia Ravikovitch (1936–2005).

The Hebrew 4th letter "D" has an angle of 90 degrees.
Four 90 degrees make a circle – that's what the haircut was about.

Four 90 degrees make a circle. That would be 360 degrees. 10 times Krypton's 36. However, four times 90 degrees also make a cross. Crosses, the number four and square angle are prominent in the Krypton proving.

Four sides, cross

On the radio, they were talking about Christ from cross to grave to sky. You need the cross. People carry their crosses all the time.

Feels as if upper torso is disconnected. Left and right across the upper part of my heart, and front and back at the lower.

There are 4 arms not joined at the centre. Joined by light, not matter.

Travelled to the underworld with the sword crossing my heart bearing all the unbearable pain.

Thoughts about the heart. Hearts are quartered like the 4 quarters of Jerusalem. Blake was talking about the fourfold division of Jerusalem – every part and thing and person is in 4 quarters.

Wrote 'cauterised' as 'quarterised'.

In my mind's eye I was seeing magic squares. I am feeling so cross.

The cross is a feature we have not yet seen in the previous nobles. It is one step further into diversity. It symbolises both the vertical connection of heaven and earth, grave and sky, as well as the horizontal disconnection, the quarterisation of the body, the heart and Jerusalem. We now carry our

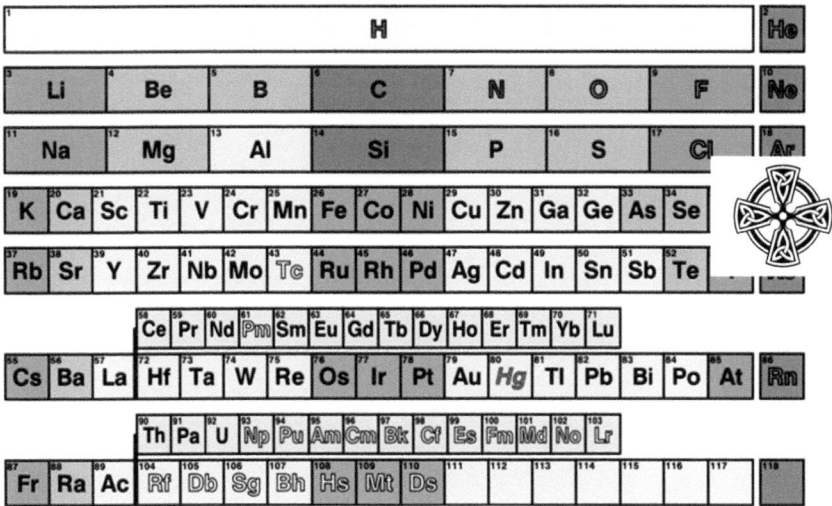

Figure 10.4 Krypton kross dissecting the periodic table

crosses, our burdens. Where we were once one, we are now four, with a square personality.

But the cross has another significance in Krypton. As I have previously mentioned, Krypton sits at the heart of the periodic table, the center point of the cross between the three nobles above and the three below. If we look at the noble-centric periodic table below, the crypton kross becomes obvious.

Squares and curves on the earth

> *An attempt at visualising the Fourth Dimension: Take a point, stretch it into*
> *a line, curl it into a circle, twist it into a sphere, and punch through the sphere.*
>
> Albert Einstein[3]

When aligned, we stand perpendicular to the earth, 90 degrees to its horizon. There will however be a 90-degree difference of alignment between those standing upright in the north pole and those on the equator, which is an important part of the following Kryptic puzzle, from the proving.

Celestial equators 90 degrees. *Plus, it in the North, and minus it in the South.* A square on the equator is a point on the pole.

Let us dissect the sentence above. The celestial equator is an imaginary projection of the equator's great circle into celestial sphere. All of its points are at 90° angle with the poles (Figure 10.5). As a result of the Earth's axial

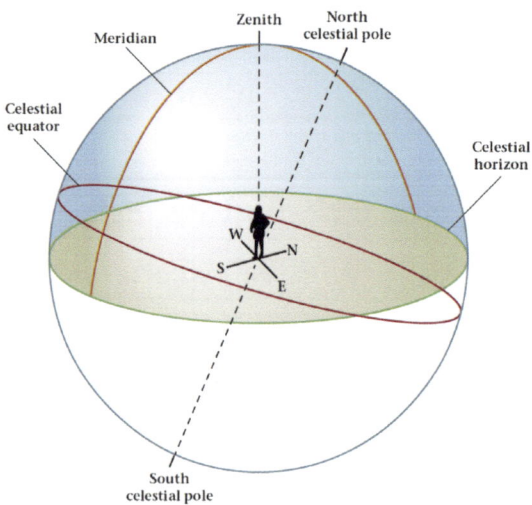

Figure 10.5 *The celestial equator and the celestial horizon*

tilt, the celestial equator is inclined by 23.4° with respect to the celestial horizon.

Plus, it in the North and minus it in the South – this is an obvious reference to the earth's magnetic field, which is tilted at 11° to the earth's rotational axis. It seems that our earth has several tilts: axial and magnetic. The earth's magnetic field arises from the earth's core, which is mostly made of liquid iron, nickel and cobalt, all of which are magnetic elements, and all of which belong to Krypton's fourth period. As these elements rotate in the centre of the earth, they produce a magnetic field, much like a dynamo.

'A square on the equator is a point on the pole'? To understand this, we must meet the longitudinal lines that dissect the earth.

Dream of using a knife to cut 4 parallel, longitudinal lines on a body.

There are 360 degrees of longitude (meridians) around the earth, each connecting the north and south pole and crossing the equator at 90°. There is no actual geographical reference to mark the beginning and end points of longitudes, unlike latitudes which relate to and begin at the equator. The international community have agreed that point zero, the prime meridian, is the one passing through the Royal Observatory in Greenwich, England (Figures 10.5 and 10.6). Hence, GMT – Greenwich Mean Time.

Dream: on parade ground in Greenwich Naval College.
Dream: I knocked on the door of a Military School (The Royal Naval College in Greenwich).

The longitudinal meridians converge at two points: the north and south poles. But the latitudes do not converge; they are parallel and stay the same distance apart everywhere. Thus, latitude signifies a distance while longitude is an angle.

A square on the equator is a point on the pole.

The angles between a longitude and latitude at the equator are square. Yet when these vertical lines meet at the poles, they form an acute angle between themselves. While there are 360 degrees of longitude, there are 24 meridians that mark the hours. They all meet at the pole. Hence, 360° divided by 24 would make the angle between them 15°, similar to the angle at the pinnacle of the letter A. Thus, the angle between a longitude and latitude is an H at the equator, and an A at the poles.

H and A are the same in mirror image.

The diagram in Figure 10.7 is a plane map projection, which is a representation of the latitudes and longitudes of a sphere placed onto a

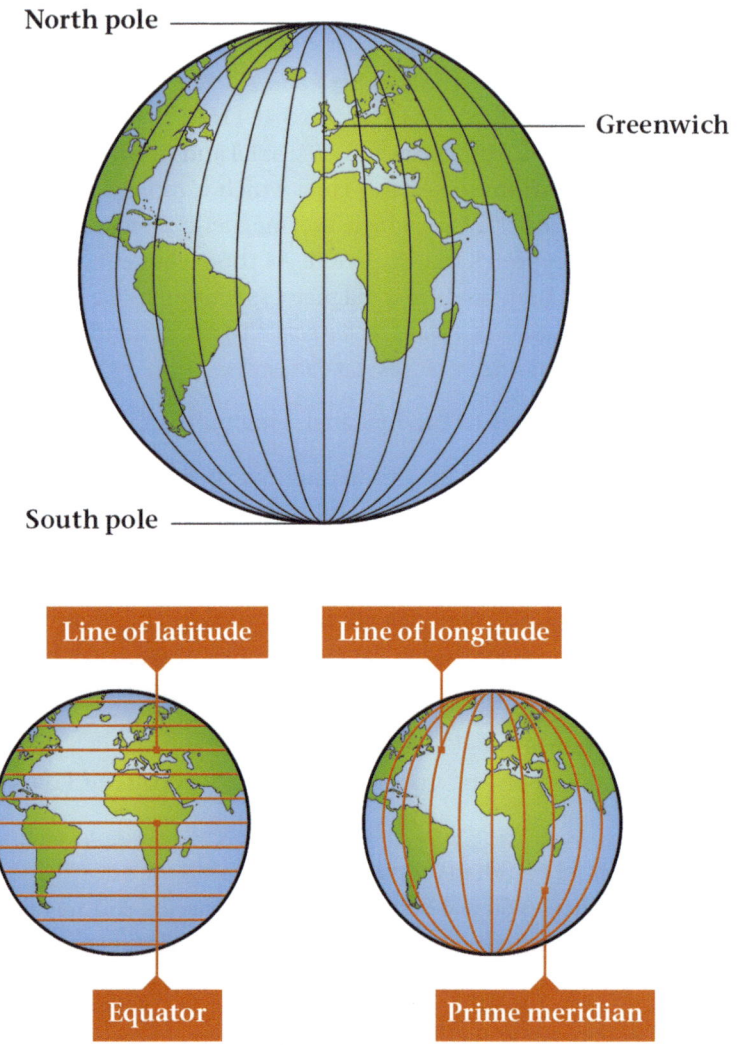

Figure 10.6 Longitudes and latitudes. Non-Euclidian geometry

two-dimensional flat surface. Map projections always distort the reality of a sphere's surface in one way or another. The two maps in Figures 10.6 and 10.7 demonstrate the difference between non-Euclidean geometry and Euclidean geometry respectively.

Euclidean geometry involves points, angles, lines, triangles etc., as drawn on a flat piece of paper.[4] Hence, it is also known as plane geometry; the stuff you learn in high school. Non-Euclidean geometry involve mainly spherical and hyperbolic geometry, which is necessary when we deal with the earth's curved surface. Spherical, as its name implies, relates to

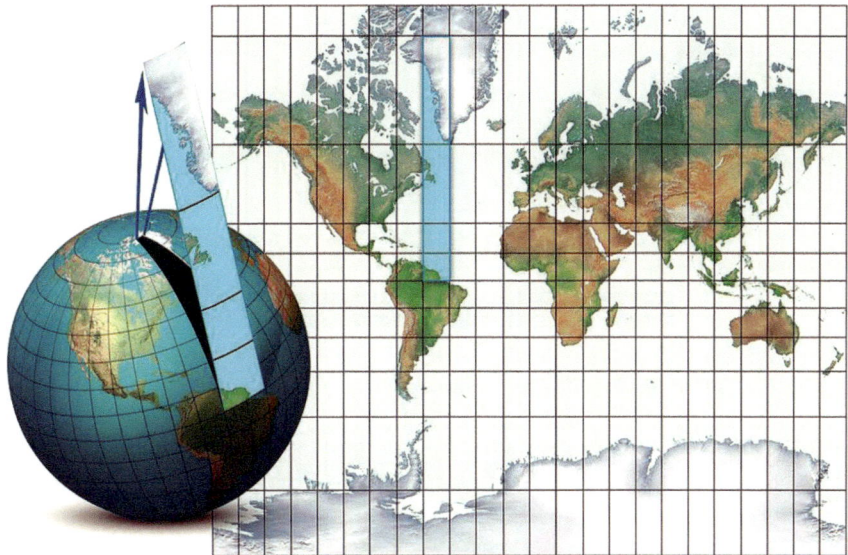

Figure 10.7 *If the earth were flat all the angles would be square. Euclidian geometry*

geometry on the surface of a sphere. It behaves differently from Euclidean or plane geometry. For instance, straight lines in spherical geometry form great circles. Triangles may have more than 180° as the sum of their angles. Parallel lines don't exist – any two lines will intersect.

A line, the first dimension, can curve into the second dimension of surface. A surface can curve into the third dimension of sphere (Figure 10.8). When a sphere curves, we get non-Euclidean geometry, curved space time. Curve the sphere and we get the fourth dimension of time (Figure 10.9).

The measuring of angles and distances between longitudes and latitudes belongs to spherical or non-Euclidean geometry.[5] While Euclidean geometry is good for architecture and to survey land, spherical geometry is essential to navigation and astronomy. Both can function in the second dimension of surface, but spherical geometry has introduced 'the curve'.

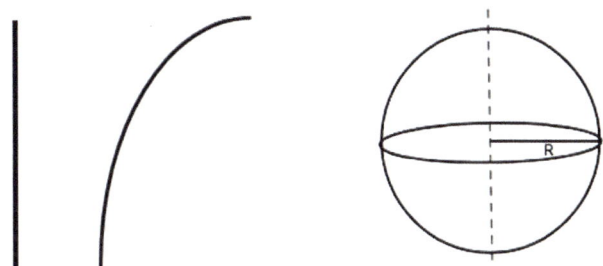

Figure 10.8 *Line curving into second dimension plane, which then curves into a 3rd dimension sphere*

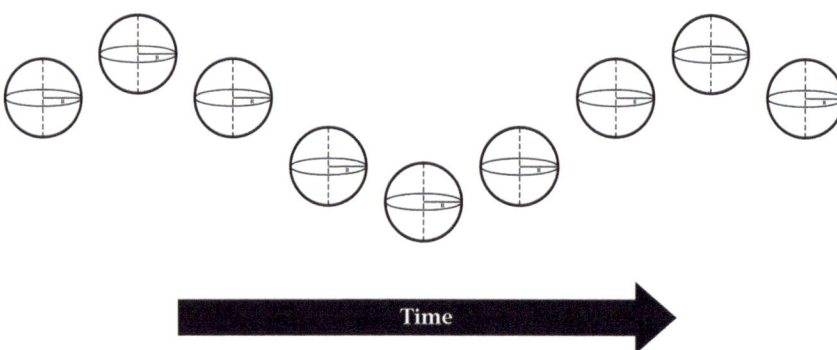

Figure 10.9 Sphere moving into fourth dimension time

Another non-Euclidean geometry is hyperbolic geometry which relates to 'curved' space and plays an important role in Einstein's general theory of relativity.

To conclude, curves can be part of the second dimension of surface (a curved line on a flat paper), but they can also curve into a ball in the third dimension (think of tying your shoelaces) or even time curving in the fourth dimension. The fourth period and its noble Krypton have moved us into the realm of curves, spheres and warped space time. And, according to physicist Stephen Hawking, warped space time may just about allow time travel.[6]

I wish I could go back in time!

In other words, the ability to change our Karma.

And herein lies the problem....

To be or to re, that is the question.

There are two opposing states of Krypton; I will call them to be – and to re –.

Be –

All I could hear was To be or not to be, that is the question, whether it is nobler mind. The words were Beheaded, Betrayed, Believed, Becalmed, Beware, Because. I was then given four definitions of what Be means: To have existence. To exist in the world of fact whether physical or mental. To become. To remain.

There was then a whole rhyme about be as a prefix. It was all about whether we becloud or whether we bedazzle. The words were beacon, beak, bean and been, bear, no bearing, beauty, beaver, beckon.

Re – Repetition

Dream I was doing the same thing repeatedly, time after time – I can't remember what.

Different chains – proton-proton – or carbon. This is to liberate us from repetition.

There was a sound like the reveille horn – or Rig Veda – to wake people up – reverberating. I feel reverend, reverence not Reverend. Revert, revere, rend, reverie. To review, a revival, I was revoked, revolving, revolutionised and rewarded. Reawakened. I've got relief.

I feel the last 30–40 years have been full of missed opportunities because I have been overcautious. Will the opportunities come round again?

Karma

My karma ran over my dogma.

Barbara Johnson[7]

The TV showed the crossing of a llama with a camel (thought they'd get a "karma") and they said they were just reconnecting evolutionary lines, but I thought that if they see time as being curved, then lines always come together anyway.

Karma is like a boomerang, and maybe a change of mind but now a change of heart.

Past family unresolved relationship clouded my day. Regret feeling for not having resolved them earlier. Intuitively perceiving that it can be restored as death is only a change of elements; another boundary, it can be accessed.

Mind tracing past meaningful experiences where I learnt lessons of the state of emotional relationship and uncovering patterns and connecting them with paths on the tree of life.

I left a banana skin on the fourth step of the stairs and thought it was funny how we create our own accidents.

Conclusion

The Geometry of Krypton take us on a ride from straight lines, square angles and crosses to curves, spheres, great circles and acute angles. It swivels us 90° from parallel latitudes to curved longitudes, the markers of time. It touches on the geometry needed for navigational and astronomical measurements, and it opens up the fourth dimension, which involves curvature of space and time.

As opposed to the first day when I wanted to stretch out, I now wanted to curve like a fossil.

This curvature, which results in spinning, is where the Krypton state become spiritually and emotionally significant. **Metaphorically speaking,** we have two extreme positions related to our location on earth. On the one hand, if we are standing at the equator, we would be at 90 degrees to the earth's axis. At this position we would spinning at a speed of 1037.5 MPH around the earth's axis. Life would re-volve.

Dream: I was doing the same thing repeatedly, time after time.

If, however we are standing at the poles, our vertex pointing north-south along the earth's axis, our own central axis would not be rotating, just being, aligned with the causeless, timeless, mindless spiritual truth of the universe.

Two doors to the world. The top one opening to the North minus reason. This is given to us, no mind all heart, freely given.

The equator position metaphorically represents the unfortunate state of Krypton being caught in a loop, riding a cycle of boredom, mental calculation, emotional replication, chronic reiteration, and karmic repetition. There would be no higher vibration, just reverberation. Life recycles with no straight line to save us from its circular trap. Every circular zero needs a one, a linear opportunity to escape its repetitive loop.

0 with 1 in the middle = ten
This is to liberate us from repetition.
I have been overcautious. Will the opportunities come round again?

It is only in the aligned polar position that we can escape the firmament of thought and belief, of repeating cyclical time created by the revolution of the earth around itself and the sun. This aligned position gives us an opening through which to exit the cycles of time. No wonder Superman's Fortress of Solitude is located in the north pole.[8]

There are still points for entering the Stargates. One of the still points is the light before dawn.

Stargates, often portrayed in sci-fi movies, are portals that allow rapid travel between distant locations in space. In New Age terminology, they represent spiritual doorways to a higher consciousness. In this context, stargates are very much reminiscent of the Neon 'window of the sky'. It is only in the Second and Fourth Days of Creation that the firmament is mentioned, and their related proving of Neon and Krypton present windows or gateways at specific vertically aligned points, portholes through which we can penetrate the barrier of starstruck rules, beliefs, concepts and logic.

The point of the light before dawn is when the sun is positioned at 90 degrees to our position on earth, a still point of stillness before we revolve into the busy day.

We may let life ride us in its repetitive cycles, or we can ride life in noble now-ness. Standing upright, at right angles to the earth, is not enough. We must learn to navigate to the spiritual poles of its axis. From re-ing to be-ing, from beheaded to becalmed, from betrayed to becoming, from review to rewarded, from the Karmic be-cause to reasonless being.

I am in a continuum present rather than in compartments of before, past, later, and so forth. I am aware of the noise that there is in silence.

However, if we do leave the tracks of our misdeeds in the sands of time, we create Karma. This can be corrected by rectification or possibly by time

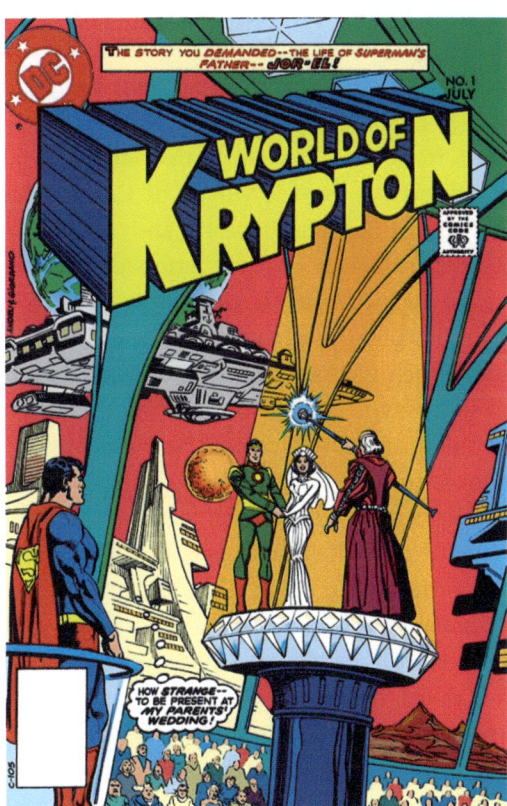

Figure 10.10 Superman curving time

travel. As mentioned before, the debate on time travel backwards to correct Karma is still open. According to Stephen Hawking it may be possible to travel back to the future but not forward to the past.[9]

I wish I could go back in time!

Dream that I went to go swimming with a friend's son who was 4. He ran off ahead. We were too early to be there and the man was not there. The child was in a hurry to incarnate. It was too early because I haven't met the man yet.

I am the mother of my father and the sister of my husband, and he is my offspring.

K or to C, that is the question.

Karnack it's not the ark but the arc – arc lights, alignments carnac.
A 'C' is a quarter of an '8'. Dismember the * and you get four Cs.

From the Greek *krypté* to the Latin *crypta*. Krypton starts with a 'K', because it is Greek (kappa) and the Greek alphabet doesn't have a 'C'. The Romans took the word from the Greek, but because they didn't really use a 'K' in their alphabet, they wrote it with a 'C', which they pronounced as a 'K'. This is how the Greek word turned into (Latin) *cryptum*, which was then used in current languages (e.g. cryptic).

From ark to arc, from the Egyptian temple at Karnack to the ancient megalithic sites around the French village of Carnac, the etymology of cryptic Krypton cross-fertilises its initial 'Ks' and 'Cs'.

It is in the geometrical shape of these letters that we see the difference of line and curve, angle and circle. 'K' can vertically align, but it also leans towards the perpendicular 90° angle of the cross and the acute angle of tilt. 'C' has the danger of being circular and hence repetitive, but its grace lies in its opening, a doorway to other worlds. Note that arc means curve. In *Helium*, the first book of this series on the Noble Gases, I promised to explain why I choose to spell Cabbala rather than Kabala.[10] Note that the spelling *Qabbala* relates to more medieval magical practices.

This should now be clear. Kabala is spelt with the letter Kof in Hebrew, which is literally more similar to 'K', but the graphic symbolism of 'C' represents the circular feminine without 'K's' sharp and perpendicular angles. The Hebrew word Cabbala means the receptive, or 'to receive', and the art of Cabbala concerns the vessel we create to receive God's light. As such the C-shaped uterus is more appropriate than 'K's' acute, angular linear attitude. However 'K' also has its Kabalistic imagery. In the Tree of Life, light does not descend in a direct vertical midline but in a zigzag fashion down the sephirot (so as not to fry us) (Figure 10.11).

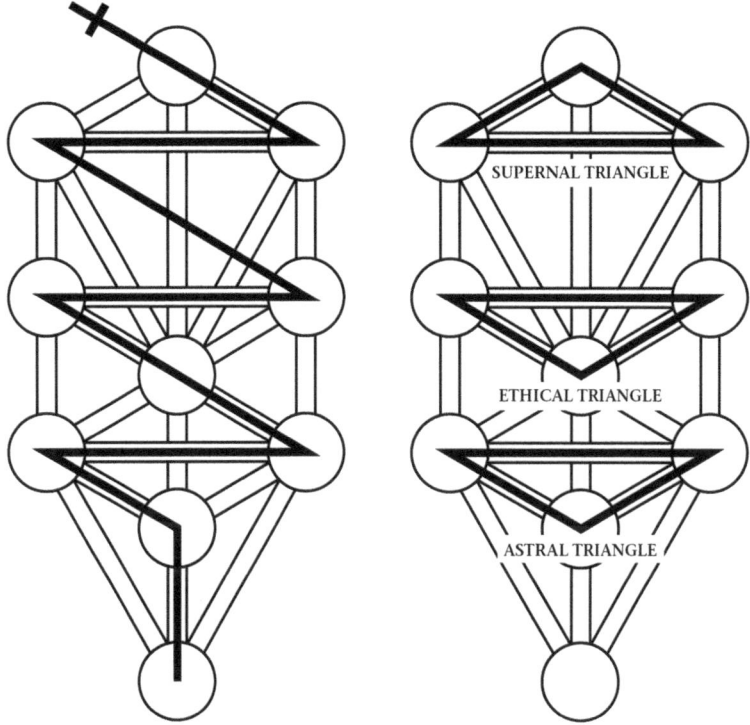

Figure 10.11 *Tree of life pathways*

Kronos and Kairos

The following are excerpts from *Creating Time*, an article by Marne Makridakis:[11]

As usual, the Greeks were ahead of us … Where we use one word to describe a whole range of things, they had the good sense to use different words to mark distinctions in reality and in experience.

Kronos (or cronos in the English spelling, from which we take our word chronology) is sequential time. Kronos is the time of clocks and calendars; it can be quantified and measured. Kronos is linear, moving inexorably out of the determinate past toward the determined future, and has no freedom. Kairos is numinous time. Kairos is a time of festivals and fantasies; it cannot be controlled or possessed. Kairos is circular, dancing back and forth, here and there, without beginning or ending, and knows no boundaries.

By contrast, Kairos was one of the subtlest gods in the Greek pantheon. He was portrayed as a winged god, dancing on a razor's edge. In one hand he held the scales of fate. He reached out with the other hand to tip those scales, altering the course of fate. Kairos was the god of lucky chance. He personified numinous moments of time giving birth to novelty and surprise.

Drawing on these ancient mythic images, we can revisit the two kinds of time with deeper understanding. Kronos is mechanistic and deterministic, time that is ruled by the dead hand of the past. Kronos devours us with remorseless certainty. Kronos turns life into stone. Kairos is creative and serendipitous. Kairos is time that is energized by the living dream of the future and presents us with unlimited possibility. Kairos turns fate into destiny.

We are not helpless to tip the balance in the direction of kairos over kronos. We can temper our fear and our fixation on sequential time. We can deepen our quest and our experiences of numinous time. In such synchronicity of kronos and kairos lies our deepest consolation and our steepest aspiration.

And from Stephen Chamberlain,[12] an English author of fantasy novels,

"What time is it?" the answer is expressed in chronological terms. But when we ask, "What is it time for?" the answer brings us closer to the meaning of kairos.

Today we live in chronological world, and the concept of kairos is all but lost. We have no equivalent word in the English language, but kairos is the notion of an appropriate time. Something is about to happen; there is an opportunity to be seized, and what we decide will affect our future. Call it the moment of truth, or carpe diem. Kairos describes the moment when the time is ripe to take destiny into our hands.

Long live the Revolution

Planets spin
Sun to shine
Mirror moon
Revolving time

Light fantastic
Beaming down
Straight or curved
Revolving time

A cause B
B breeds see
Repeat again
Revolving time

My brain reflects
A heart not mine
Disconnect
Revolving time

Karma dogma
On my mind
Digital
Revolving time

Evolution, revolution
Cyclical design
Tomorrow is my yesterday
Today's revolving time

References

1   Pearce JC. *The Crack in the Cosmic Egg: New Constructs of Mind and Reason* Rochester VT: Park Street Press, 1971, p76. Available online at: http://tinyurl.com/yrrpwh38 (accessed July 18, 2023).

2   Simon and Garfunkel. *Slip Slidin' Away.* Track 11 on album *The Concert in Central Park* (Warner Bros, 1982).

3   Einstein A. Available online at: http://tinyurl.com/2rhydbyz (accessed July 18, 2023).

4   Artmann E. Euclidian Geometry. *Britannica.* Available online at: http://tinyurl.com/3b5ryxcn (accessed July 17, 2023).

5   Introduction to Non-Euclidian Geometry. *Math & the Art of MC Escher.* Available online at: http://tinyurl.com/pm3tbpre (accessed July 17, 2023).

6   Hawking S. Space and Time Warps. *Academic Lecture,* 1999. Available online at: http://tinyurl.com/3fsxemc7 (accessed July 17th, 2023).

7   Johnson B. *Barbara Johnson Quotes.* Available online at: http://tinyurl.com/mp-pvru4m (accessed July 17th, 2023).

8   Fortress of Solitude. *Wikipedia.* Available online at: http://tinyurl.com/ytvjwmfb (accessed July 17, 2023).

9   Hawking, S. Space and Time Warps. *Academic Lecture,* 1999. Available online at: http://tinyurl.com/3fsxemc7 (accessed July 17th, 2023).

10 Sherr J. *A Dynamic Materia Medica – Helium.* Glasgow: Saltire Books, 2013.

11 Makridakis MK. Excerpts from article, *Creating Time. Creativity Portal.* Available online at: http://tinyurl.com/yc64fn7z (accessed July 17, 2023). *(Permission from author to use quotes.)*

12 Chamberlain S. Chronos and Kairos, the Gods of Time. Available online at: http://tinyurl.com/8wftsbxb (accessed January 7, 2019).

11

KRYPTON CM: NEW DIMENSIONS

A mind that is stretched by a new experience can never go back to its old dimensions.

Oliver Wendell Holmes, Sr[1]

Great knowledge sees all in one. Small knowledge breaks down into the many.

Zhuangzi[2]

It takes a genius to perceive the fifth (or eleventh)
dimension.
A scientist may understand the fourth,
a revolutionary concept.
Most of us exist in the comfortable confines of
3-D, believing this to be
reality.
An infantile can live a plane life in the second dimension
and never know better.
A moron can survive in the first,
toeing the line.
But only the Holy One, blessed be He
can manifest one dimension
out of nothing.

When it comes to dimensions, there are several different points of view, from Bosonic string theory to superstring to M-theory and more, with the number of space-time dimensions stated as 10, 11 or 26. That knowledge is beyond the scope of this book. My aim is to scan and simplify the subject and present a few thoughts of my own. However, thanks to 30 years of research, I do have an advantage by way of knowledge previously unavailable. i.e., the noble provings, their correspondence to the dimensions and the seven days of creations. These are the ideas I want to share. It would be useful to you to have read my previous books on the noble gases.

The more evolved and developed our mind is, the more dimensions we can perceive. The novel *Flatland*[3] tells of first dimensional beings stuck in a line, who can never imagine the second dimension, and of the more evolved second dimension people existing in a superficial surface, who cannot perceive the third dimension, much like a 'skeptic' who cannot comprehend homoeopathy. As we evolve, 3-D people seek to penetrate the conceptual barriers into the fourth dimension and beyond.

Historically, the earlier Euclidean[4] theory perceives three dimensions of space, and a fourth dimension in time. This concept is outdated. Let's move one step beyond. According to Rob Braynton's video and book, *Imagining the Tenth Dimension*, the first three dimensions occur in space: line-space, surface-space, and sphere-space. The next three dimensions are in time: line-time, surface-time, and sphere-time.[5] According to this model, the fourth dimension is line-time, duration, or a 'time continuum', i.e., a linear chronological progression stretching from past to future. If we continue this line of thought, the fifth dimension is two-dimensional time, time on a surface, freed from its confining line so that it can spread in several directions or circle back to choose alternate possibilities where any sequence of events becomes possible. The sixth dimension is sphere time, in which we are free to travel to 'any-time-place' instantly. In the seventh dimension, you have access to the possible worlds that start with different initial conditions. Similar thoughts maybe be read in phys.org.[6]

However, this concept is also somewhat partial, as time and space are intrinsically linked. One cannot conceive a line extending through space without it also going through time. In 1848, Edgar Allan Poe was the first to propose that 'space and duration are one.[7] Hermann Minkowski, a Polish mathematician and teacher of Albert Einstein, first put the idea of spacetime into mathematical theory,[8] and Einstein fully established it in his theory of Special Relativity.[9]

So now, rather than the previous idea of space and time manifesting separately, we will look at perspectives in which space-time manifest together in each dimension.

Thus, each of the physical dimensions contains time within it, and time unfolds into higher dimensions just as space does. There is 0-D dot time, 1-D line time, 2-D plane time, 3-D sphere time, and 4-D continuum time (Figure 11.3).

Based on the analogies between the noble provings and the unfolding periodic table, Krypton relates to the fourth dimension. Understanding 4-D can be quite complex, but the revolving Krypton brain loves this kind of complexity.

The fourth dimension is difficult for us to understand because we live in a three-dimensional world. Well, actually, we don't, but you believed me for a moment, and that is the point. We have 3D consciousness, and that is what limits our perception. A flatlander living in a surface would have great difficulty in understanding our three-dimensional world. Think of a

Figure 11.1 *Time as a continuum in 4-D above, versus our 3-dimensional view of time below*

playing card trying to grasp the concept of an elephant. The card would only see paper-thin cross- sections of the elephant as it walks by, thin lines growing bigger and smaller. This is how our three-dimensional conscious-ness perceives 4th dimension time. Thus, we only see cross-sections of time's 4-D continuum as it passes through our world, so that it seems like a movie jumping from one frame to another. From our limited third-dimension perspective we freeze time's continuous flow into frames, like a black and white film (Figure 11.1).

> *It is the insertion of man with his limited life span that transforms the continuously flowing stream of sheer change ... into time as we know it.*
> Hannah Arend[10]

Notice how in the Krypton proving, provers are transformed into the fourth dimension. Very cool.

The concept of time has changed. It feels more as a continuum present rather than in compartments of before, past, later, and so forth. Very conscious about the present moment, continuum present.

As if not really in touch with time, not really knowing what time it was, while normally I think 'I have to go to bed at this hour or that hour' and then going to bed. Now it was as if time wasn't really existing. As if time runs through my fingers. No matter what I do, I can't get a grip of things or time. It just slips through my hands.

A present infinite, a present that is always present, it's never past or future or anything.

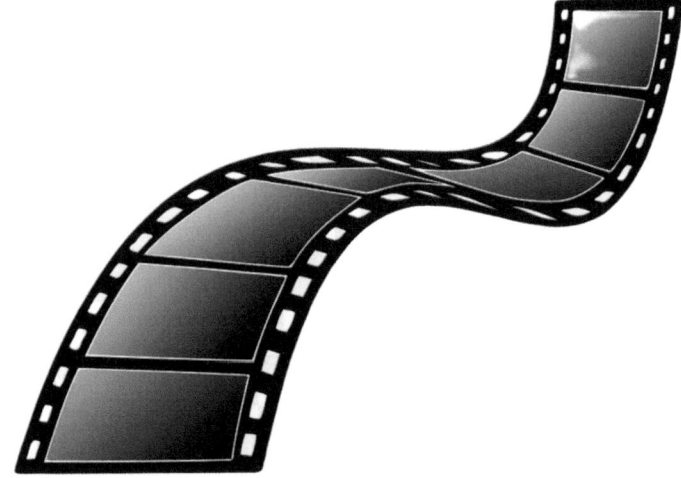

Figure 11.2 Our 4D life from a 3D perspective

I recommend that you watch YouTube movies explaining the fourth dimension, as these can illustrate the concept better than two dimensional images.[11] Drawing the fourth dimension on paper is challenging, as paper is in the second dimension. Nevertheless, Figure 11.3 is an attempted 2-D representation of the first four dimensions.

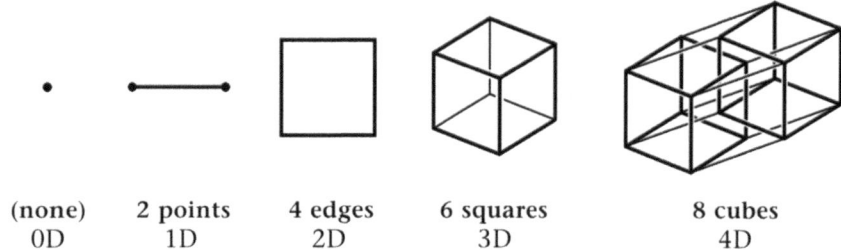

(none)	2 points	4 edges	6 squares	8 cubes
0D	1D	2D	3D	4D

Figure 11.3 Four dimensions drawn on 2D paper

Each dimension has 2^n vertices (corners or end points). A dot has none 2^0, a line has $2 = 2^1$, a square plane has $4 = 2^2$, a cube has $8 = 2^3$. Therefore, a hypercube has $16 = 2^4$. As you can see in the line contains 2 points, a square 4 lines, a cube 6 squares and hypercube 8 cubes. If this is confusing to you, at least you now know how a Krypton's mind may think.

Mind bending evolution

Let us now discuss how each dimension evolves into the next. In Figure 11.4 we can see each dimension creating the next one by replicating

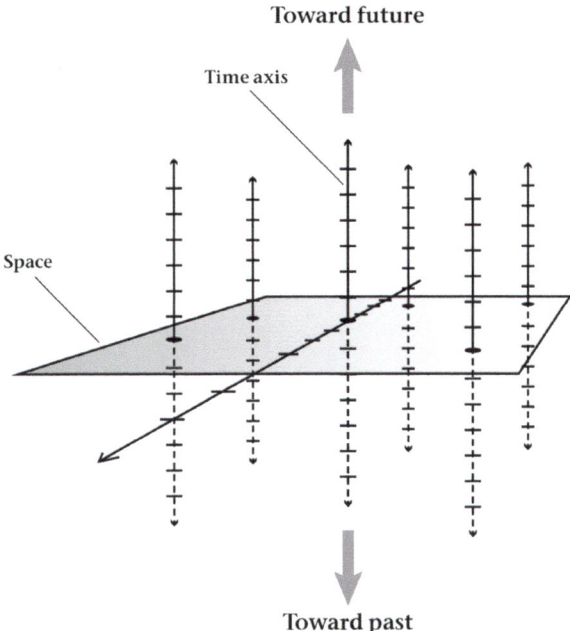

Figure 11.4 *Each Dimension creates the next one by replicating in perpendicular*

perpendicular to itself. Many dots extended into a row to create a line, many lines in parallel create a plane and many planes lying on top of one another create a cube.

Taking this idea one step further, according to some theories, time might lie in a direction perpendicular to space (Figure 11.5).

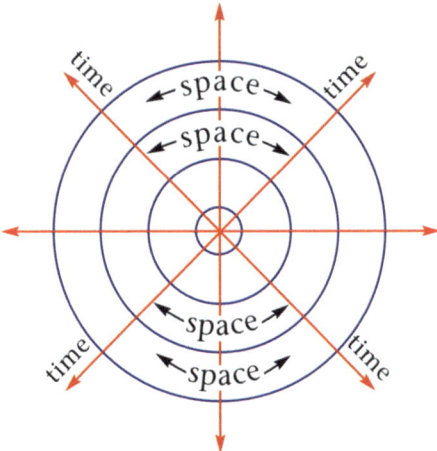

Figure 11.5 *Time perpendicular to space*

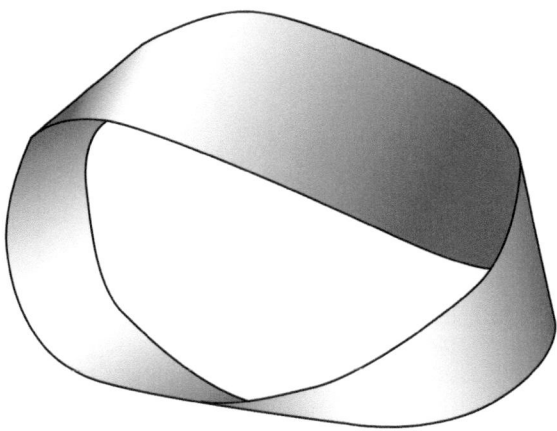

Figure 11.6 *Möbius strip*

Another way to evolve from one dimension to another is to curve or fold it. A line will curve into the second dimension of plane, and a plane will curve into the third dimension of cube. Fold a line into a circle and you get a surface. Now fold a flat newspaper into a tube. There, you have a 3-D object. This is the principle of a Möbius strip, where a 2D strip of paper is curved into 3-D (Figure 11.6). Many works of speculative fiction feature a plot structure based on the Möbius strip, of events that repeat with a twist.[12]

From this we understand that a cube or sphere will move into the fourth dimension once it begins to curve. As I have mentioned before in this book, it is the curvature of spacetime by matter that creates gravity, and 4D time (Figure 11.7).

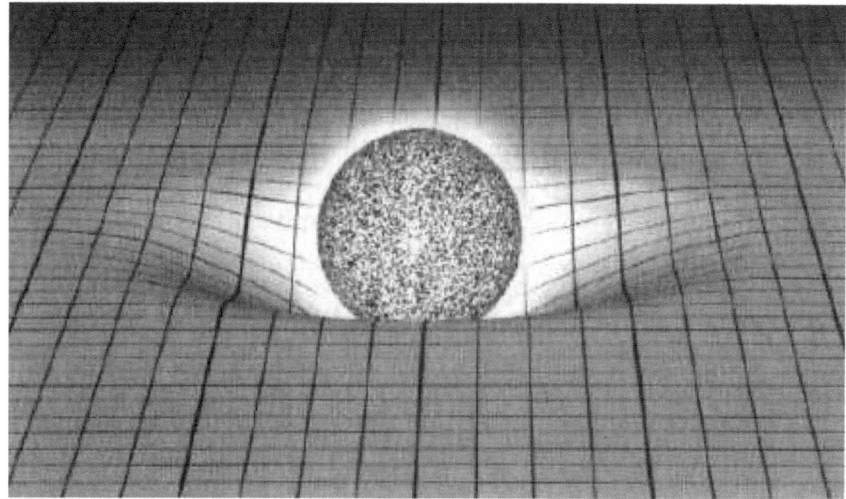

Figure 11.7 *Spacetime curving to create gravity*

On the fourth day
God created the curve
And the curve brought forth
stars, moon, sun
spinning, cycling, marking time

So as to create these
heavenly bodies
all God needed
was to initiate gravity

When gravity was introduced
matter coalesced into planets
stars fused, galaxies swirled
black holes tempted red dwarfs.

To create gravity
all God needed
was to warp spacetime.

God leaned forward and
with one finger
imperceptibly
touched the firmament.
Spacetime curved
gravity pulled
light bent; time coiled
planets formed
intellects measured themselves.

God
created the multiverse
with the minimum dose

How does this curve originate? One theory states that each dimension has an infinitely small curve within, so that it very slowly unfolds into the next dimension. As the curves develop, a line will curve into a second-dimension circle and a surface will curl into a third-dimension tube.

Another possibility (my thought) is that rather than the curve existing all through a dimension, it is there in potential but only begins to manifest once a dimension is fully unfolded and stretched to its utmost capacity. Think of a rubber band stretched in a line to infinity. It will begin to curve due to underlying curved spacetime. Likewise, only when a plane has stretched to its full capability does it begins to bend into the next dimension of cube. One can see this curve beginning to develop as we approach the end of a period. Here is gallium met, element 31, approaching krypton's 36:

Noticing every curve of the terrain. This diagram came up in my head, a circle and a point in the center. Boarding a plane which had to circle around and around. A large circle on the outside. People are sitting in a circle.

Here are Helium and Xenon curving into the next dimension, after reaching the full capacity of the previous one:

The air was so fast, it was starting to curve round. (Helium)
Air moves faster over curve, up lift like over wing. It was very large, a big room with a crescent curve in it. The people were taken halfway to the equator due to the curve that there was on shore. (Xenon)

The Eddington experiment[13]

On May 29, 1919, British astronomers Dyson and Eddington set out on two expeditions, one to the West African island of Príncipe, and the other to the Brazilian town of Sobral. The aim of the expeditions was to measure the gravitational deflection of starlight passing near the Sun. Newton saw gravity as the force between two objects, while Einstein viewed it as a curve in spacetime. Of the two most likely outcomes – 0.87 arcseconds from Newton's theory and 1.75 arcseconds from Einstein's theory – the results were closer to 1.75 arcseconds. "Einstein Theory Triumphs" was a headline in *The New York Times*. The main idea of general relativity is that mass causes spacetime to curve. If an object moves in a straight line in spacetime, and the spacetime through which it moves is curved, then the path of the object from a distant perspective will appear curved.

Noble provings, dimensions and the days of creation

In the previous three books of the Noble Gases series, *Helium*, *Neon* and *Argon*, I described the striking relationship between the first three nobles, the three physical dimensions, and the related analogies concealed within the Biblical story of creation. Here is a brief recap.

Helium is stuck in a line, with the simple decision of whether to descend; to incarnate or to remain in the world above. The Helium patient rigidly clings to the upper realms, standing upright and refusing to tilt into the world or get involved in a messy, dirty, dangerous life. In the first day of creation, pure light is created, its linear beam extending on forever, or at least until it reaches a black hole that will tempt it to curve. Once Helium does eventually bend, the second dimension of plane begins to unfold, and with it the second period, beginning with lithium and culminating in the Neon surface or firmament.

The second period unfolds a second-dimension flat surface. Neon is trapped in this surface, living the superficial and naive life of a supine, horizontal baby: I drink, I pee, I itch, I scratch, I want, I get. But it does not have the depth to see others or to form emotional relationships with them. From provings and clinical experience I have found that remedies on the second period are two dimensional and horizontal, lacking the third dimensional spine necessary for standing upright (e.g., Beryllium, Boron, Oxygen). In the biblical creation story, we find the flat firmament of day two (represented by the ozone layer), and water's flat surface everywhere (H2O). Once Neon's second dimensional plane fully extends its surface potential, it begins to curve, like the ocean. Like a sheet of paper pulled too far, surface begins curling into the third dimension. The biblical waters now concentrate in one place, revealing the earth.

The third dimension is introduced in day three, as mountains and trees stretch skywards and throw shadows upon the ground. These are the emotional aspects that develop throughout childhood and teens, allowing us to discover our shadow side and to form meaningful relationships. Hence remedies from this period tackle the issues of discovering their identities (e.g., Alumina, Phosphorus and Sulphur), or growing a spine (Silica). Our crawling baby has developed a spine and identity and can now stand on his own two feet and see the other. This day presents fruits and seeds, the procreation born of adult relationships.

Only after the third dimension of volume of sphere is fully unfolded in Argon can it warp into the fourth-dimension of time-space, manifesting the fourth day's gravity, sun, moon, stars, and seasons. In other words, definable, measurable time. Argon's timeless garden of childhood curves into the office clock.

You may wonder how this reflects on a Krypton patient. One aspect is that there may be a conflict between segmented time frames that compartmentalise one's life causing fragmentation, dismemberment, and disconnection, as opposed to the spiritual state of a time continuum. Gravity, the daily grind, and Karma also demonstrate the curved time of Krypton.

Returning to the way dimensions unfold, yet one more idea (me again, based on the provings) is. I should say that this is my own theory for which I have found no scientific backing. Yet that the development of temporal dimensions lags the spatial dimensions by one. In dimension zero, the dot, there is no time.[14] In the first dimension of line, time is still in dot phase, entanglement, where all things happen simultaneously (noticeable in the Helium proving, as in seeing the double of a same person at once). Surface or plane develop a linear time of simple past and future, a one directional arrow of time, as can be seen in the Neon proving. The third dimension of sphere displays surface time, as in the Argon world of our childhood: we are vaguely aware that 'time' exists, but it loiters and lingers, holding no particular significance. Summers stretch on forever, and who cares what time school starts and when bedtime is. Time is superficial to us, not integral. Here is Krypton harking back to Argon's childhood.

I get absorbed in activities losing sense of time and end up being late for appointments. Reminds me of being a child and being absorbed in playing.

I'm losing it, time is deluding me. Important stuff is becoming unimportant and unimportant things take on great importance and big dimensions.

Once we move into the fourth dimension, time curves and revolves in a sphere, we put on watches and set alarm clocks to become responsible adults, the prisoners of time. We become time.

I will illustrate this idea with the following table and some quotes from the provings.

TABLE 11.1   Temporal dimensions versus spatial dimensions

Dimension	Space	Time	Space phenomena	Time phenomena	Noble gas	Day of creation
0-D	Dot	None	Singularity	Pre-Creation, no time		Day one 1st part Chaos
1-D	Line	Dot	Light	Entanglement, one time	Helium	Day one 2nd part Let there be light
2-D	Plane	Line	Flatland	Past – future	Neon	Day two and Day three 1st half Firmament and water curving into land
3-D	Sphere	Plane	Geometry	Childhood time	Argon	Day three 2nd half Grow vertical trees
4-D	Warped sphere	Sphere	Gravity	Wake up time	Krypton	Day four Sphere curves into cyclical time

Here are some examples from the respective provings:

Helium:

Dream: Another time than ours, it stretched across different centuries.... A bear-hunter came.... He was wearing a thick, bearskin coat. He came from the outside, was a stranger, kind of timeless. He belonged to any time, but he was also very present in the actual time at the moment. He could fit into any time, but was himself whatever time he moved in and he was always respected as himself.

Neon:

Time is moving relentlessly and remorselessly forward, and I'm stuck behind, unable to keep up. Prior to taking the remedy, I felt too far in the future without realizing it. I feel as if I have taken a step back and am in the here and now.

Argon:

My time sense is totally gone. I have no concept of hours, days, or weeks. It could be any amount of time since the proving started. It is as if time didn't exist.

Krypton:

As I curled up and as I stayed there, I went through the ages of time.

In the next book of this series, Xenon, there is a probability that we will meet the fifth dimension, surface time, the unfolding of life's multiple simultaneous possibilities.

I have problems with numbers, especially 5s.

Radon, in the sixth dimension will allow time to cube. Prepare to blow your mind.

A final diagram to represent the information above:

The double helix gyre of Krypton would create the mirror image principle as it appears in the proving.

I was witnessing the birth of letters, seeing them coming into being in English and Hebrew. Hebrew starts at the back of the book.

H and A are the same in mirror image.

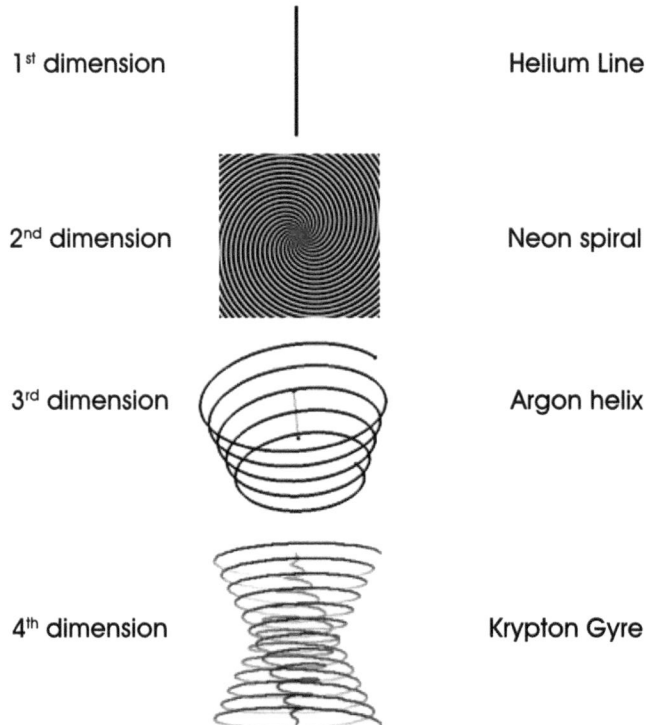

1st dimension   Helium Line

2nd dimension   Neon spiral

3rd dimension   Argon helix

4th dimension   Krypton Gyre

Figure 11.8 *Development of spacetime structure in different dimensions*

You can study these concepts further in the Kabbalah by Leonora Leet (1929–2004).[15] Leonora was a Professor of English at St. John's University and the author of *The Universal Kabbalah, The Kabbalah of the Soul, Renewing the Covenant,* and *The Secret Doctrine of the Kabbalah.*

The periodic slide – new dimension
(To be read in a Dr. Zeus rhythm).

No- thing was every-where
No-thing was every-time.
No-thing was bored.
No-thing decided to pack up its no-things
And go no-where else
But it left some-thing:
A dot

•

Dot was every-thing
Everything was dot.
Dot looked around.
There was no-thing to be seen
Dot tried to move up.
Dot tried to move sideways.
Dot tried to move forward.
It could not. It was dot.
Man, this was frustrating
Dot could not take this for much longer.
Dot got all en-tangled with itself
The pressure was building, fast
Dot was getting mad, real mad
Dot was about to expl-!

Bang.

Dot was free!
It was heaven, it was bliss
One-thing it was not;
Dot became a No-Dot.

Dot expanded
Up, down, back, forward, sideways,
For a million billion whatevers
Dot pushed its own envelope
Expanding into the No-Nothing
which remained
After No-thing split.

Now No-Dot was Not-Now
And No-Dot was Not-Here
No-Dot had moved somewhere
Between then and there

It rolled and expanded
At incredible pace
Till Not-Now became time
And Not-Here became space

But No-dot was scattered
Battered and shattered
Finding direction
Was all that now mattered

Because No-Dot was lost
And it looked all around,
No-One to be seen
Not even a sound

It longed for direction
A place to call home
And it wished that no-thing
Would pick up the phone

It wished that no-thing
Would drop it a line
Just then No-thing called
I hope all is fine?

Here is your line
It's called 'I-me-mine'
Please confine to this line
That leads from up down.

A line? That was fine
I will slide down this line
That extends from mid-heaven
Into some-body's spine

In a golden shrine
On top of cloud nine
Line waited its turn
Line bided its time

Photons forged atoms
Helium fused sun
Light banished dark
End of day one

But Line became fixed
Compulsive, Obsessive
Line would not bend
This got quite excessive

Dirty or clean
False or be true
There was really no way
Of combining the two

Two? You said two?
Knock knock! Two of Who?
Two dimensions, it's us
And were saying to you –

Line, Look through the keyhole
And see what is new
Break out of your shell
Line, Find the true you.

Set yourself free
I will lend you my strength
Take a step sideways
Curve out of length

More space to play in
Sheet, surface, square
Combine length and width
There is much power^2 there.

You can tilt to the future
Lean to the past
Scratch till it itches
Reach for the stars.

Well width's what I long for!
Thought line with a sigh
I'm tired of floating
T'ween mud and sky

I need a good stretch
He said with a yawn
I'm bored of this prison
and feeling forlorn

I'm needing to flex
And I'm longing to bend
Time to grow wide now
Time to extend

Tired of this axis
Heaven and earth
I'm taking the plunge
I'm going to give birth!

Line took a step forward
Took a step back
Opened the doorway
Heard the shell crack

Oxygen grasping
Hydrogen's two
Ozone dividing
Second day through

Time twisted and curled
Space was a whirl
Universe dancing
Galaxies swirl

And a star fell from heaven
Split into two
And he looked at his mom
And he said hi what's new?

Now a baby's a baby
Until it grows ripe
It functions quite simply
It works like a pipe;

You pump food in one side
Some love and a drink
And it comes out the other
With quite a big stink

It cries and demands
It screams till it gets
It doesn't see others
It doesn't care yet

There're some babies I know
That at age forty two
Can't get satisfaction
And scream till they're blue

So, to reach for the stars
Or melt into bliss
They shoot up some junk
Or just take the piss

It's a shallow existence
Of joy, discontent
So we're longing for depth
To give us a vent

As we float in our ark
Side by side, two by two
It's time that we turned
And recognized you.

We'll send out a dove
Open our throat
Find some expression
Get off this old boat

Find us some earth
Let waters recede
Search for some soil
In which to plant seed

Earth will grow grasses
Earth will sprout trees
Play in the garden
Happy and free

It was time to gain height
It was time to gain depth
Take a step sideways
Time to have sex!

And OOOOH sex felt good
And OHH Sex felt nice
No wonder Day three
Was declared 'it's good' twice!

What makes sex so special?
The X I am told
Meiosis crossover
So life can unfold

But when surface is cubed[3]
From paper to tube
When flat becomes thick
There's a chance for lovesick

For a puppy love youth
And a child's fairytale
Can't go on forever
Without getting stale

When childhood is over
And lovers are gone
When youth's glow has faded
It's time to move on

Can't live my whole life
Like an old Peter Pan
Time to grow up now
Evolve into man

Evolve or revolve sir?
A question of time
Grandfather clock
Or digital line?

You want to grow up?
Well, spin time around
Get a career
Work daily grind

Moon circle earth
Earth circle sun
Recycling time
Is the end of all fun

Wake up at seven
Home around five
Repeat the next day
Just a way to survive

Live in the moment
or bear karma's cross
life is eternal
or life can be dross

Aliens visit
In slick UFOs
Geeks recite mantras
Buddhas crack codes

Crossing the mirror
Things ain't what they seem
Kali to Krypton
Stages eighteen

Heart beats to minute
seventy two
that's twice thirty six, sir
and nine times eight too

From not to dot to line to square
To cube and into time
Each fulfilling a new aspect
Each another rhyme

A song of great dimensions
One two three and four
The question we are asking now is
Are there any more?

To be continued....

References

1 Holmes Jnr OW. *Wikiquote.* Available online at http://tinyurl.com/msby9vyw (accessed July 18, 2023).

2 Zhhuangz. *Quotefancy Zhhuangz Quotes.* Available online at: http://tinyurl.com/ ywxk2p6h (accessed July 18, 2023).

3 See: Abbot EH. *Flatland: A Romance of Many Dimensions,* 1899, and Sherr J, *Dynamic Materia Medica of the Noble Gases, Neon.* Glasgow: Saltire Books, 2015.

4 Space-time. *Wikipedia.* Available online at: http://tinyurl.com/2w74ba44 (assessed July 17, 2023).

5 R Bryanton. Imagining the Tenth Dimension: A new way of thinking about time and space. *Goodreads.* Available online at: http://tinyurl.com/yut7pebr (accessed July 17, 2023).

6 Williams M. A Universe of 10 Dimensions. *Universe Today,* December 11, 2014. Available online at: *Phys Org:* http://tinyurl.com/2hhudvvy (accessed July 18, 2023).

7 Horgan J. Did Edgar Allan Poe Forsee Modern Physics and Cosmology? *Scientific American,* Jan 24, 2015. Available online at: http://tinyurl.com/2bws2yre (accessed July 19, 2023).

8 Galison P. Minkowski's Space-Time: From Visual Thinking to the Absolute World. Available online at: http://tinyurl.com/yckaspmj (accessed July 18, 2023).

9 Overduin J. *Gravity Probe B.* Einstein's Space Time. Available online at: http:// tinyurl.com/55tuen5d (accessed July 17, 2023).

10 Arendt H. What's Changing? – Time. 2023. *Halcyon.* Available online at http:// tinyurl.com/3hzs6xus (accessed July 18, 2023).

11 Bryanton R. Imagining the 10th dimension. *You Tube.* http://tinyurl.com/ kuy4mtpj (accessed July 17, 2023).

12 Möbius strip. *Wikipedia.* Available online at: http://tinyurl.com/2s3hrthh (accessed July 17, 2023).

13 Britton J. Eddington's Eclipse Experiment: 1919 and 2017. *The Naked Scientists,* May 29, 2019. Available online at: http://tinyurl.com/ah9nmuhc (accessed July 18, 2023).

14 Sherr J. *Dynamic Materia Medica: The Noble Gases: Neon.* Glasgow: Saltire Books, 2013. Chapter 10, pp68–78.

15 Leet L. *The Secret Doctrine of the Kabbalah: Recovering the Key to Hebraic Sacred Science* and *The Kabbalah of the Soul: The Transformative Psychology and Practices of Jewish Mysticism.* Rochester VT: Inner Traditions Bear and Company. (Original edition 16 November, 1999.)

12

KRYPTON SYNTHESIS
OF PART ONE

The following is a synthesis of Krypton, based on sensations and functions, or the *verb* of the remedy. Please note that sensation and function are interchangeable and form a cycle.[1] You can switch and mix sensation and functions. Play around. All the expressions below are inseparable and make one totality.

Sensation: Connected
Function: Disconnected

Sensation: Continuous time
Function: Fragmented time

Sensation: Continuous present moment
Function: Caught in a time loop

Sensation: – Tall, high up, mountains
Function: Slip sliding downwards, gravity

Sensation: Straight line, aligned
Function: – Must curve

Sensation: Magnet, gravity
Function: Must curve

Sensation: Energy flowing
Function: Cut off, disconnected

Sensation: Cut off, disconnected, blocked, no flow, can't move forward
Function: Must re-verse and rotate

Sensation: Rotating
Function: Must recycle

---

[1] For more information on this method of synthesis, please see Sherr J., *Dynamic Materia Medica: Syphilis*, Saltire, 2012.

Sensation: Reversal
Function: Mirror image

Sensation: Mirror image
Function: Must decode

Sensation: Emotions cut off, heartless
Function: Recycle intellect

Sensation: Cut off from God
Function: Intellectual spirituality

Sensation: One
Function: Four

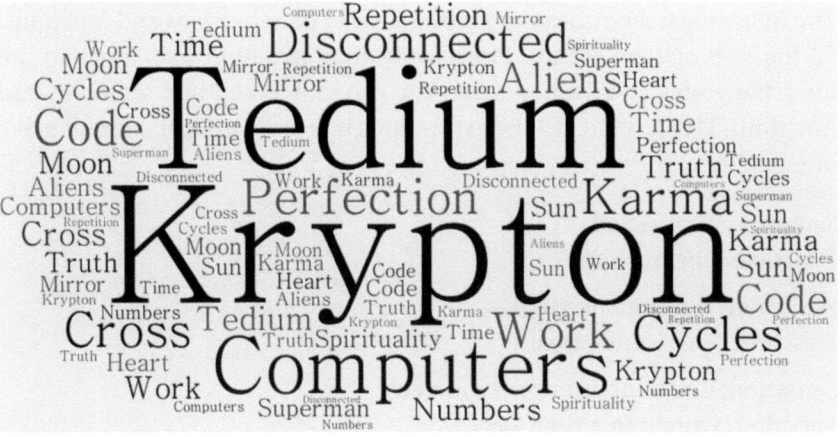

Figure 12.1 *Word of Art.* Available online at: https://wordart.com/ (accessed April 28, 2024)

Adjectives: Turning, bored, tired, weary, curve, turn round, repeating

Nouns: Sky, galaxies, planets, sun, moon, time, aliens, UFO's, mirror, code, hieroglyphics, numbers, mathematics, cross, Superman, Tarzan, hero, animal power, drugs, perfection, truth, intellect, academia, mundane work, treadmill, Karma, repetition, spirituality, computers, worthless, guilt, head off

Image: Modern man – *homo Kronos*. Life on a treadmill. Recycled intellect.

> I went to work work work work
> I had had a reasonable day day day day
> At work work work work work.
> Now I am home
> But no one is there

Chakra: Heart
Day of creation: Fourth
Colour: Green
Musical scale: F
Dimension: Fourth, linear-curved time
Whammy: Intellect, work, profession
Book: *The Little Prince, Cryptonomicon* by Neil Stephenson
Movies: *Groundhog Day, Superman I, A Beautiful Mind*

13

KRYPTON CASES

I am particularly pleased with the following Krypton cases which illuminate and confirm many aspects of this remedy.

In the previous books in this series, I have included quite a few cases from other homoeopaths. However, I have received only three Krypton cases from my wife and two from Dynamis graduates. You have to know this remedy to prescribe it, but once you do, the cases are out there!

Note: I have marked essential words or expressions that indicate Krypton in **bold.**

CASE 13.1 'I come from another galaxy'

Homoeopath: Jeremy Sherr, UK

Female, age 64, born 8 March 1958

Background
Patient has been off work with depression. Her main complaint is a **"totally destructive body clock"**.

Consultation
*[Patient arrives 40 minutes **late** for the consultation.]*
    P: The letter said 12 and I know we said 11 on the phone but then I should have known it takes half an hour to get here from Paddington. (Laughs).
    *Observation: **Scruffy looking**, dirty old pullover, herpetic eruption on mouth and lips which she scratches all the time.*
    P: I've previously taken many remedies, much Sulphur, Nux-vomica and others. Everyone gives me Sulphur.
    I've been off work with depression for a lot of time. I'm still off work but I convinced the company doctor that I'm fit enough to go back to work on a part-time basis.
    I have a tendency to viral infections. At the beginning of the year, I had two months off work with a cold/flu-type virus. At the moment, my main problem is **a totally disruptive body clock**, which means that I don't fall asleep until 6 or 7 in the morning.
    Dental abscesses. A big problem is I've got cold sores all over my face.
    I suffer from backache, which at the moment isn't constant, so that's actually improved.
    My depression is all work-related cause I feel I'm being bullied by the company. I've got to pull myself together and start taking legal action against them because they are taking disciplinary procedure against me due to bad attendance, because I was forever going off sick with all these viral infections. I'm allowed so many absences in a certain period otherwise I'm kicked out. But now I'm out with depression. I was first diagnosed with depression about 10 years ago when I had problems at work as well. Then I was off from work last summer; then I was alright for about 6 weeks; and it's been **going downhill** ever since. I think it's possibly more anxiety than depression because

every time I think I'm fit enough to go to work, **I think about going to work, I just feel ill. I just can't face going to work.**

Can you explain that?

P: It's like a kid's thing, sort of where they don't want to go to school 'cause they are being bullied. I just get a sick feeling in the pit of my stomach.

Depression. It's been around for a long time?

Yeah.

What's the main feeling of it?

The main problem I've got is tiredness. Initially when it started, it was tearfulness, but that's gone now. I think as far as I'm concerned, it's sort of sleeping problems.

But what is the main emotional feeling with depression?

A sort of lethargy, **I sort of feel numb**, I feel like a zombie (laughs).

What is your work?

I work as an **analyst programmer – computers.**

And how do you feel about your work?

Well, the actual work is fine because I joined a new department in August. I wasn't happy where I was before because I was just **too bored**, and they couldn't understand when I said I want to move because I felt too **stressed out through boredom.**

What do you mean "by boredom", can you explain?

Well, work that is **not mentally challenging enough.**

Can you tell me about your work, what you like, what you don't like, what bothers you, what doesn't?

I like sorting out problems where I've got to think, analyze. Someone says "Right, this program isn't doing what it's supposed to be doing, find out what's wrong with it".

And what kind of work don't you like, what aggravates you the most with work?

Well, I don't even mind doing **mundane stuff**, but when you're doing it **week-in week-out** and work that someone says "Right, do this bit of work. **It should take you a week,"** and I do it in 5 **minutes** and it's working fine. I can't be bothered to do anything a lot of the time. Lack of energy, I'd say. And problems sleeping.

Ok. And emotionally?

Emotionally it's just the lethargy, **nothing affects me** (laughs).

Is there anything that makes you feel better?

Oh yeah, when I get an agency ringing me up about **a possible new job** (laughs).

I've got certain skills that I can use well, doing it **beats half-heartedly**, but also at the moment because I've had so much time off sick, I don't think anyone would be prepared to employ me.

I'm very easy-going, but I hate fussy people (smiles).

What do you mean, fussy?

Everyone has their own things that are important, but people who get **wound up** by what I see as trivial things.

For instance, what things are trivial?

The way they look, or you know, **if they've got a hair out of place or a little spot of dirt on their clothes.**

I don't like being controlled and I generally don't control others. I can't see why human beings need to control each other. **Sometimes I wonder if I'm from this planet at all (laughs). I don't understand human beings.**

What do you mean, can you explain that?

Well, I can't understand the way human beings behave towards each other sometimes.

So, what planet do you think you're from?

I don't know.

Where?

I don't know, some unknown planet, **maybe another galaxy.**

A galaxy?

Yeah.

That far away?

A-ha.

Which galaxy?

I don't know, I don't know what they are all called.

I do believe in instant karma. If you do something nasty to someone, then that same thing, something nasty will happen to you kind of thing.

Instantly?

Hum, fairly soon. Well, sometimes it happens in a lifetime, because **I believe in reincarnation as well.** You're sort of **reincarnated to address your past mistakes kind of thing.** But I do find that sometimes I can't understand how they can do that or whatever, then **I turn around** and do the same thing myself (laughs).

I've got strong affinities with Mexico, **ancient Mexican cultures**. Mayan, Aztec-like.

Right. You work with the green party?

Well, that's in my so-called free time (laughs).

And what are the environmental issues, what is the issue that gets to you the most, what aggravates you the most?

I think it's what people are **doing to this planet**.

I like doing cryptic crosswords, logic puzzles.

What do you mean?

Things that **involve using the brain**. You get like a magazine and it says "5 people each went shopping on a different day and what colour jumper did each wear?" and you get various clues to that. Like so and so went shopping the day before the person with the red jumper, but the day after the person who bought the packet of biscuits", or something like that. From **the clues** you get, you've got to establish who went shopping on which day, and what colour jumper they were wearing when they went shopping, and what they bought.

Mathematical or just logic?

Logical. But I do like mathematical calculations because I'm pretty good at maths as well.

What kind of things?

I like logical puzzle books which had mainly numerical puzzles in them or crosswords. You've got to work out what the numbers. They give you the **clues are in sort of algebra** formats, and you've got to work out what the value of each letter is, and it goes into crosswords puzzle grids, so you've got to do a bit of math's calculations.

My weaknesses are that I hate writing documentation (laughs). But sometimes, having said that, I'm a bit of a **perfectionist** and sometimes I spend more time writing documentation than the actual work is going to take.

When I was small, my mother used to send me and my brother off to school **last minute** so we wouldn't get into mischief. When I used to go to church with my parents, we'd usually leave at the last minute and end up **turning up late there**. But also, some friends that I go out with now, we arrange to meet at a certain time, but once you get to know people, you know they're not going to **turn up on time**. So, you think, "Well, there's no point in me **turning up on time**, I'll just be sitting there on my own". So quite often I turn up half an hour late to meet my friends and I'll be the first one there (laughs).

I feel better when I am **somewhere on time**. Also journeys, things like that. Flying somewhere I tend to **turn up on time**. So when it's really important, I turn **up on time**. If I didn't turn up at such and such time the train would leave; whereas if I didn't turn up at work on such and such time, the work would still be there an hour later.

I program computers in **C language**.

For what kind of programs?

For an airline, **scheduling aircrafts**. So, if they want to fly from A to B they've got to work whether there is a suitable aircraft available and make sure that all the flight plans and everything, that the aircrafts are where they are supposed to be for the next part of the journey.

That sounds like a logic puzzle?

Yes.

What's your favorite number?

Thirteen.

Remarkably, the patient's name is Astra! The star.

Rx Krypton 12C, for 13 days

Follow-up two 6 weeks later

Observation: Big smile on her face. Her hair looks blacker, eyes more blue, and cold sores around her mouth are gone. She is dressed more neatly.

So how have you been generally?

I've been very well, my general health and my mental health have improved. I did have a sort of viral infection recently.

What changes have you noticed?

I feel more energetic and less lethargic.

Your mental health has changed?

Yes, I feel much happier. More ready to get involved in campaigns and things.

More involved?

Yes. A lot more positive outlook on life, on my future and all that. Especially about getting a new job, more positive.

Good. The depression?

That's generally gone. I feel OK at the moment. I want to get involved in physical exercise and get back into cycling, which I haven't done properly in about 10 years.

Your sleep, apart from the arm, how is it? [She had phoned about some arm pain that prevents sleep]

Apart from the arm, it's generally OK. My sleep patterns were totally up the creek, so before, a lot of the time I wasn't getting to sleep until about 6 in the morning, but now I go to bed at about 1 o'clock and wake up around 6.30–8.00 o'clock so it's a reasonable sleep pattern.

Normal hours rather than the 6–12?

Yes, now it's gone.

How is the phlegm in the throat?

That's OK, better but still there but probably because I smoke (laughs).

Has it improved?

Yes.

Herpes? Backache?

All gone. Only this shoulder pain that I had a long time ago seems to have come back. Now that prevents me sleeping instead of my clock.

How many percent better would you say you are, generally?

I'd probably say 80 to 90%.

Great. Do you still think you're from another planet?

Oh, that's right (smiles). I think so (laughs). Maybe everyone else is from another planet. Instant karma keeps hitting me in the face. A lot of time I think, "How can people do that?" and then I'll **turn around** and do it myself. You gave me Krypton didn't you? Isn't that superman?

Are you doing puzzles and that kind of thing?

Yeah, but I'm not as obsessive as I was. Before I would pick up a puzzle book, especially when I was off work and didn't have to get up, and I'd sit there for at least 5 hours doing puzzles. Now I might do a little bit of puzzles, but I do other stuff as well.

I feel a lot better than I did before. Before I had depression, but I kind of came out of it. I feel better, I feel I can cope with life in general (smiles).

Patient continued to do well as long as I saw her for a couple of years, with repetition of Krypton 12C when needed.

Jeremy's comments

I find this case to be remarkable as it fits Krypton so very well. Her body clock is out of time. Her frequent expressions of "turning up", "turning round", or being "wound up" demonstrate the revolving aspect of Krypton. The depression is typical to this remedy as it is the result of boredom and lack of mental challenge at work, resulting in an emotional numbness. Her love of logic and math puzzles, the belief in karma, as well as the profession of being a programmer scheduling air traffic are all typical of this remedy. It was interesting to learn of her attraction to Mayan and Aztec cultures, who were also star gazers and have much in common with ancient Egyptians. The cherry on the cake is her being from another galaxy, and of course her starry name: Astra. I gave Krypton 12C for 13 days because of her affinity for numbers and the number 13. I thought she would like that. She did.

CASE 13.2 Stuck in a rut

Homoeopath: Camilla Sherr, Israel

Male, age 34

Consultation
I'm depressed, **stuck in a rut**. I hate my job. It's a **repetitive** factory job. I have to constantly smoke dope to control it. I'm angry, I lose my temper, it's ridiculous.

Everything is jaded, there's **no sense of wonder**, I don't get excited about anything. I feel like everybody is conspiring against me to make me feel like this. It's very difficult to get up in the morning. I was very nervous about coming, it's hard to talk to people I don't know. I never feel happy, the only way I can control my moods is smoking dope, that way I'm not ranting and raving. I'm in a volatile relationship, competitive with my girlfriend, it's easier to argue if I'm stoned. I'm ok walking on the hills, but as soon as I come down, I feel bad again.

I always want to be outside the system. I didn't want to work, to become a **slave** to the capitalist system, but here I am, stuck in something I don't want to be. I'm very cynical. I have a degree in sociology. I hate exploitation. I never wanted to get a job in the system, now I'm like one of those people I used to hate, **not realising my full potential**. I'm not fulfilling expectations. I went to private schools, and now I'm just working in a shit factory polluting the environment. I'm a socialist.

I have **no motivation**. I need to get out to a **job that is more fulfilling**. I'm so busy, working overtime, stressed at small things, stupid things, they piss me off to the extreme. I think that people are going to judge me, you're going to think I'm a really horrible person.

My upbringing was good, private school, degree in sociology, that's where things stopped, I tried to do a PhD but I didn't complete it. I don't **like not completing things**; in fact, I have a fear of doing things in case I don't manage to complete them. **I hate being late**, it's disrespectful. I had years of not doing anything, just travelling. I have the weight of the world on my shoulders, I'd just like to wake up one morning and be happy.

I have a lot of guilt about events from the past, trouble I got myself and other in to as a teenager. I took loads of different drugs. I smoke cigarettes, I just can't stop. I was naughty as a kid, hated authority, I was an anarchist. I tell bosses to fuck off, they abuse their position, I'm on a crusade against evil management. Capitalists have no respect for people as individuals. It's the **monotony of the work**, so **repetitive**. I dwell on things, I get obsessed with things. I would love to live in India as a **spiritual man**, I'm into **Buddhist philosophy**. I love music, I get obsessed with things, I've got to have this mobile phone, this video. I think a lot about money. I actually make more money from my current job than I would be making as a social worker. I get bad hangovers from very little alcohol.

I have spine problems and my neck is out to the side, it feels as if the right side of the shoulder is up and out of shape, worse moving my head to the right.

I just fell into this job, I'd like to be working with homeless kids, I love kids, I get on with them great.

Allocating time is difficult for me, I've got to do something all the time. I do either everything at the same time, or nothing at all. I am a shift-worker. Even if I work from 3 pm to midnight I force myself to get up at 8 am, or else I get really angry with myself. **I have to be on time**, I hate being late. I am **cynical and constantly analysing** everything.

My girlfriend and I are constantly trying to prove the other one wrong.

Rx: Krypton 200C, twice

Follow-up after two months
I don't know if anything happened, but people around me say I'm more pleasant to be with. I'm calmer. Right after taking the remedy I felt "trippy". I'm happier, but that's because I changed my role at work, I have a new role at work now which is not as boring or repetitive. I have also cut down on dope significantly, I hardly smoke at all. I don't feel I need to do everything at the same time like before when I did 100 things on a day off, which used to stress me out. I don't do that anymore.

My neck was much better, now it's playing up a bit because in this new job, I'm sitting down all the time bending forward, this gives me a bad posture, I prefer standing up. It feels weird and twisted, one day the pain is on one side, the next day on the other side. My headaches were almost gone, I only had one last Friday due to drinking a lot and got an unbelievable hangover.

I'm getting on with my girlfriend a lot better. The only issue is that she does not want kids and I do. My sense of time is better. It has been a lot easier to wake up lately, and I don't give myself a hard time if I don't get up at 8. I'm also much less cynical.

What about the feeling that nothing is worthwhile and not getting excited about anything?
Did I say that?

What about everybody conspiring against you?
[Blank stare] I don't remember saying that either. No, I don't feel that at all.

What about wanting to be outside the system?
Actually, I haven't thought about that at all since taking the remedy. It was about taking responsibility and finances. I don't feel like I'm kicking against the system so much now.

Weight of the world on your shoulders?
Did I say that?? I'm doing the union work and it seems easier. [He launches into a long speech about how the situation is very difficult from the management point of view, and how he can understand their difficulties as well!]

Obsessed about things?
Like what?? [He doesn't remember saying that.] No, I don't do that.

How about the guilt feelings?
He replies he hasn't thought about it once.

Rx: repeat Krypton 200C, when needed
He continued to do well until last seen after one year.

Jeremy's comments
This case has the typical hallmarks of Krypton: Repetitive work, boredom, ennui, issues around time, and being late, the feeling of being stuck in a rut with yearning for spiritual freedom, and the tendency to over-analyze. The feeling of not fulfilling one's potential, and the fear of not completing things are typical of noble gases), as is the obsessive nature.

We can learn more about Krypton from this case. On one hand: socialist and anti-capitalist tendencies, work-related issues, feelings of being a slave; but on the other hand: thoughts of money. The cynicism is typical of people whose intellect overrides their heart. The affinity for kids and the longing to laugh innocently are a craving for the Argon state of childhood. These issues may lead to the excessive drug use, which in this case has been clinically helped. In the follow-up, we see another characteristic of the nobles, which is aggravation from bending and amelioration from standing.

CASE 13.3 Tarzan

Homoeopath: Jeremy Sherr, USA

Male, age 60
I am a lecturing professor of literature. Previous homoeopathic treatment was Aurum, Lycopodium, Nux-vomica, Stannum metallicum, and Phosphorus, which helped a little.

Consultation
The patient is depressed and has low energy. He suffers from chronic fatigue, drags around and feels he **isn't fulfilling his potential**.

He had an operation on his left shoulder.

He suffers from bad back pain, due to stress. He has pain in his left shoulder socket and thigh, which are worse for strain, like swimming, and worse from thinking about them.

Twenty years ago, his marriage went on the rocks. He wanted to become a freelance author, but it never happened. He was under a lot of pressure and stress.

"I slipped into 1960s sex fantasies, smoking lots of dope, cheap hotels. I was traveling in **Mexico** looking for **spiritual shamanic teaching.**"

"I fell short of performance. I couldn't keep up."

He had a back injury with a lot of pain, worse from his kids jumping on his back.

He says "**I've not come up to my responsibilities**. I ruined the kids' vacation and disappointed them." He has lots of **guilt**. "The responsibility is a burden, it's too much for me. The kids ride on my back".

The dope aggravated him because he was worse from smoking. He has difficult respiration, worse from exertion. He has a cough which is worse from stress and tiredness. His expiration is difficult.

He began intense bouts of medication, but it all felt heavy and dense. 100 things to think of a second, 100 things to visualise. He became very depressed. He feels **heavy and dense, has no fun**. He has to **do his duty, has his nose to the grindstone all the time**. There is **no joy in his life**. He just **lives his life mechanically**, going to work every day – each day is just another day.

He feels great **despair – has no bliss**. Has to **work hard because so many things go backwards**. When he started to work on his book, he broke his hip and never got any further. He lost the whole book with a **hard drive crash**. "It broke me."

He has blown both shoulder joints because he tried to swim faster than his friends. He has to work harder than anyone else, but has nothing to show for it.

There's always something going wrong, so he tries to **work harder and faster**, to swim harder, but his friends would just go further and faster without trying.

He began getting seriously into **tantric Buddhism**.

He is depressed – he says he **"works like a dog"**, **"like a beaver"** and **"like an animal"**. He believes he was crucified in past lives. His muscles are weak, his oxygen is low, and his libido is low.

He says, "as a child, **I felt like Tarzan** and used to pretend I was Tarzan". He used to jump from one tree to another. But one time when he tried, he fell on his stomach and was surprised.

As a child, he used to get cramps in his abdomen.

He developed whooping cough during his wedding ceremony and also before orgasm.

He is very sensitive to smells.

He has nightmares about **missing buses and planes**, which cause anxiety. He has anticipatory anxiety and **he is always late**.

He is much worse from the cold, and he has a lack of vital heat.

Cold and damp especially make him worse.

He suffers somewhat from tachycardia.

He has been going into the **mountains to practice Tibetan Buddhism** and says, "**I've worked very hard at meditation** for the past 20 years."

Rx: Krypton 30C, one dose

Follow-up three months later
Generally, he feels much better. "I feel clearer and more focused – I **now finish things and accomplish more and am much happier with my work**."

His back pain is gone. He used to have to go to the chiropractor every three weeks but now has stopped going as there's no pain. His tendonitis is also much better; he feels less restriction.

"Before I used to injure myself whenever I exercised, but now I can go ahead without hurting myself, I manage my body much better".

"Also, my breathing is stronger, I can swim, and train and I oxygenate much better. There's no fatigue when I exercise, no difficulty breathing; no more obstacles to doing what I want to do!"

The repetitive strain pains in his hand, wrist and elbow are much better. "I can work on the keyboard all day without any problem – I'm free! Free to type as much as I want, without any restrictions."

His mental focus and concentration are also much better. "I can cut through obstacles. Whereas I used to procrastinate if something slowed down a project or became an obstacle, now I just do it! My procrastination used to be my biggest block. I can concentrate for longer **because I now allow myself to play in between**. I don't approach it like a task I have to gird my loins for. **I fool around a bit**,

write a bit, play a bit; then because I play, I work happily and don't stop so I'm very happy with work. I'm just finishing writing a university book".

"Because I'm more involved in what I do, I get much more **joy from my work – it is now my fun!** I get satisfaction from it".

He's also taken on new initiatives. "I volunteer more for things. I now feel I have the resources and am more available. I want to pay back for what I've been given!!"

He feels he has much more self-respect. "I'm more forthright with people, I state my mind more openly, say what I think, and am more relaxed with my colleagues. I expect more respect and value for my work!

"I now feel very happy and am spending money on new clothes. I've also designed a new room for my work and computer. I've had a change of values – I can spend money on myself which I never felt able to do before. Before, I only ever gave to others, **I felt I should work hard so the kids have money. Now, I'm the kid!"**

Rx: Krypton 30c, when needed

Jeremy's comments
This patient was on a treadmill leading to nowhere. Once again, we see the Krypton themes of unfulfilled and unsatisfying work, over-responsibility and guilt. "With nose to the grindstone", He "works like a beaver". Each day is just another day, and work is mechanical. Interestingly, he repeats the same expression from the previous case of "100 things to do". The lack of joy leads to an escape into spirituality, fantasy and drugs. Paradoxically, he even "works hard" at meditation. As in the previous case (Case 2) we see a man not fulfilling his potential. This is similar to Helium, but rather than a soul mission is more career based. This is the second case with affinity to South American spirituality.

What is important in this case is that we see the other side – Tarzan flying from tree to tree, much like superman, but in leopard-skin cloths. Unfortunately, he misses and falls on his face. Hence, the recurrence of expressions such as "I fell into" or "I slipped into", and everything going backwards.

Very typical of Krypton are the dreams of missing planes, as well as losing all one's work in a computer crash. I should know.

This is the third case in which we see with back pains and left [?] shoulder problems, all related to the heavy burden of work and responsibility. As in the previous cases, there are respiratory problems. This patient also has the tachycardia that fits Krypton's heart affinity.

His final comments that "work involves play and play involves work", and that "now I'm the kid", show a healthy harmony between child and adult.

CASE 13.4 Mirror mind. Stroke from overwork

Homoeopath: Jeremy Sherr, Tanzania

Male, age 54

Background
This patient is Sigsbert Rwegasira, the "Tanzanian homoeopath", who introduced homoeopathy to Tanzania and made it legal through indefatigable efforts. I allow myself to disclose his name because he is no longer with us today, and it is important he is remembered. From my friendship and knowledge of him, I believe he would not mind.

Sigsbert was tall, upright, calm, charismatic and good looking, with a twinkle in the eye. He came from a noble family, a royal lineage of one of the most intelligent tribes of Tanzania. He was a chemical engineer, but suffered from severe malaria bouts since childhood. After he was cured by a passing homoeopath, he raised money and travelled to the UK to study homoeopathy. He opened the first clinic in Tanzania, and after initially being harassed by the authorities, managed to convince the health ministry by means of his excellent results. Working alongside the ministry, he passed the *2002 Tanzania Alternative and Traditional Medicine Act*, legalising all forms of alternative medicine.

His clinic was always crowded. He treated over 200 patients a day, mainly with malaria. Through his brilliant mind and with much practical research, he developed an excellent combination remedy for malaria, using rare remedies, which works very well even in the most difficult cases. He had begun establishing a homoeopathic school, but never completed the mission.

Sigsbert was a noble person, intelligent, charming, with a strong tendency to overwork. His patients loved him and depended on him. He had a deep understanding of esoteric matters, which is quite unusual in Tanzania. He was a good friend. I used to fondly call him Ziggy Stardust.

Sigsbert had been severely overworked for many years. I and others warned him, but he would not stop. Six days a week he would get up at 4 am, drive two hours to work and finish at 8 pm, then drive the two hours home. On the seventh, he would lock himself in a room, read and do mathematical puzzles.

Consultation

At the time I saw him he had suffered a second stroke in 18 months. Hypertension was the cause, and it had affected his life and health badly. He could no longer work. He had taken many homoeopathic remedies with little help. Here is his remarkable case.

"If I get stressed, my blood pressure goes up, my heart beats fast and I feel tense in my head, with palpitation and difficult breathing. Then I must relax for a while."

He has not been well since the stroke. "I have become sleepy during the day, never had it before. I get very drowsy and want to doze off". He is putting on weight, has loss of memory, difficult concentration, sleepiness, and visual problems.

Reading is difficult since the stroke. His vision is distorted. "If I look at the number 50 I see 500."

"I used to write a lot, I love writing, but since the stroke, I don't want to write, it is too big a task for my brain. I have become a lazy writer, no drive. I can't sit in one place for long anymore".

"After the stroke, my right-hand side was affected. I began seeing an image of a car coming from right side is coming towards me, very disturbing. I can no longer drive, and I can't work."

"When I read a paper, I miss stuff on the right. When I want to lift a pen on the right, I hold it upside down".

He has some heart burn, with severe burning pain in stomach, worse from wheat.

"With the high blood pressure, I had pain in the heart and pressure in head".

He has some herpes simplex in the corner of his mouth.

His eyes are yellow brown since childhood, maybe caused by a weak liver from quinine and malaria. He had pain in his liver in the past with malaria.

Since his stroke, he has a strong desire for raw onion.

He desires olives intensely.

He has an aversion to nuts and salt.

Coffee causes high blood pressure.

"I am vegetarian to calm down my mind. **I over think**".

"I have a strong passion for animals, would never hurt an animal".

He tells me about the high vibration rate of animal protein, from a study and from his own understanding.

"I practice meditation". (At that time unusual for a Tanzanian.)

He has many **dreams of flying**; he flies very well and is in control.

"I am clairvoyant, since 1993 when I began meditation, I hate this, it gives me a pain in the eyes. It began with a peculiar sensation that **my third eye flipped and turned inside out**. It revolved 180 degrees. After this, I started seeing the aura colours of people".

"If I see a person's top half only, like when they are behind a table, **I see the shadow too**, as if seeing though the table, the non-physical shadow, a faint bottom-half image. **I see the bottom half of anything that is hidden**, like an arm behind a curtain. It is involuntary. When I pay more attention, it disappears".

"When I give a lecture, if someone has an idea, I see a flash of yellow coming out of their vertex even before they say anything. I see lines of energy down meridians".

"If I want a solution to something, the flash comes in my mind. I try to avoid this, I don't like to just know things. I can get a flash or a sign of the solution, like an intuition, and it will be right".

"My mother was psychic, but I am not fascinated by it".

When my third eye, flipped it was **like seeing the universe upside down**, with an inward pressure pulling my eyes in. It would happen involuntarily".

"I **would see inside out**, like you think you are looking from the outside, like a **new vision**. I want to tell people what I see, but they will think I am crazy. If you see what people are not seeing, **you are in a different dimension**. It is upside down or inside out, but more than that, **I can't explain it. Because others have never seen that**".

"It is like seeing a human aura, when a person moves, I see a soft jelly-like colour moving along with him. It is as if someone **flipped**

or reversed the switch in my mind. When it happens, I am glued down and don't feel like moving – a shock, and I can't think. A total change of perception. Somehow, I came out of the normal way of viewing things and the world is different".

"I grew up in poverty. When you grow up and come out of it, part of you remains there, and you compare. If I see people living that kind of life now, **I want to bring them to the other side.** I am very generous, give a lot of money".

"I joke a lot; it is a weakness and a strength. I make friends easily, crack jokes".

"I like children, but have no time for them".

"I used to be reserved, never raised my hand in class, but it changed with time" (hand turning over rotating inside out).

"If someone annoys me, I don't get angry but I speak out, **tell them straight, tell the truth".**

"I am **not a people person, I don't want to mix in parties or meetings,** I don't go out. I lock myself in my room and read; I am more comfortable if I'm not disturbed".

"I was a good reader, **I love philosophy, things that make the mind digest,** not easy reading.

"I **work very hard, too many hours**; it is my nature, but also life here in Tanzania. On my one day off, I lock myself in a room and do **maths and logic puzzles.** I love that. Otherwise, I **read philosophy and esoteric books which I love.** I love to **be alone and read, I spent too little time with my kids".**

Rx: Krypton 30c one dose, repeat when needed

Follow-up two months later
"Very good improvement all round. My energy is back, drowsiness is gone. I can work again. Memory and concentration are much better. The images of a car coming from the right have gone. The heart pain is much less, and my blood pressure has reduced".

The visual disturbance since the stroke is just about gone, and I no longer miss stuff in my right field of vision. I am less obsessed with maths puzzles and spent a bit more time with kids. I can read and write again. The main thing is I am back to work!"

He remained well over the next 18 months with occasional repetition of the remedy, but fell back into overworking, partly due to external pressure and local circumstance, and partly through his dedication to patients, the huge demand for his service and his addiction to overworking. Perhaps also the money, he had come from poverty. He just couldn't stop working. Two years later he suffered a massive stroke which incapacitated him, and nine months after that he passed away.

Jeremy's comment

Sigsbert's noble nature and upright stature, the keen intelligence, the desire to be alone, the tendency to overwork and the love of maths puzzles and esoteric books are all indicative of Krypton. The need to tell the truth is also typical of the nobles.

More important, however, are the strange rare and peculiar features of this case, ones which he had both before and after the stroke. These features fit the proving of Krypton very well. It seems that through meditation something transformed in his "third eye". This is the exact point Camilla highlighted in her proving. His third eye not only opened but "inverted", as if turning inwards. From then on, he moves into another dimension, which is difficult to describe, but it is something of a mirror image of reality. He can see upside down and inside out. His inner eye has the ability to create a whole image out of half an image. Like Superman, he has x-ray vision and can see under tables.

Exactly the opposite happens after the stroke, where his mind is not able to see half the images, though it still manufactures vision from the right. Of course, these symptoms are quite common after strokes.

Locked in his room and mind, his frontal brain revolved. It seems that the involution of the third eye transported Sigsbert through the Kryptic mirror and into the other side, to a new, perhaps fourth dimension.

We miss you, Ziggy Stardust!

CASE 13.5 ET go home

Homoeopath: Jeremy Sherr, USA

Male, age 49

Consultation

From his wife: He's a pilot, he was in the Air Force. He's a very conservative guy, **not emotional**, says what he feels, stays in the background. He worked in radar. During his work with radar, he **monitored a UFO**, after which he went missing for 2 days. He has no memory at all of what happened during this time. He starts crying when he talks about it. He has never been well since; he is very upset.

After this episode, he lost a lot of memory. Usually, he doesn't cry. But he was so scared that he became **paralyzed** with terror. He will just repeat, "I can't talk about it, I'm paralyzed with terror".

He is obsessed with UFO's, obsessed with the universe, and with Stephen Hawking.

Space is so vast. How do they get from here to there? He freaks out from the size of the universe. He thinks of life beyond the universe, how people traveled. Is there life outside the solar system?

He has a sense of righteousness and truth. **He never lies!!!** He says people should be honest. Humans on earth are a gross species. A comet should hit the earth, it would be a great thing **to start over**. People can't be trusted.

He sits quietly, observes, and analyzes, He sees everything, knows everything in his environment. He is so aware of what he does, so aware and **so meticulous**. He is an airplane mechanic; everyone trusts their lives with him.

He is an incredible pilot, very **cool in an emergency**. If an engine fails at 300 feet, anyone else would want to jump. But he is so cool. Extremely cool in an emergency. He is the person you want. **A Hero!**

But **never lie to him or be untruthful**. If you do, you are out of his life, he doesn't forget it.

He is a very deep feeling person, gets very hurt.

He is a great guy. He sits up all night feeding abandoned kittens. He is a devoted good guy, yet feels human beings should be destroyed, maybe by a comet or anthrax. People are so disgusting, they destroy the ecology, not honest, no integrity.

He has anger and resentment inside.

He is a quiet, sullen man; but if he trusts you, he is the life of party, funny. Great sense of humor. He will never turn you down.

If he is your friend, he will give you his car or his shirt.

He **loves flying, it becomes him. He is a bird**. Any airplane suits him. He is completely fearless in storms and difficult situations. Flying is his passion.

He is an only son. His father and mother were strict and unfair.

He doesn't go out with the guys. He doesn't relate to men; he fits in with women better.

He is a very **responsible man**. "You can't let the kids fall".

From the patient:

"I was born on a farm, all my life on a farm. I was not shown love. "Do your chores". I had wonderful parents, but not affectionate.

I never studied, but got good grades. **I am intolerant of imperfection. I see a fault and dislike it**. I hate if something doesn't work right and is supposed to.

If it didn't go right, I would smash it and buy another one.

I always fixed machines. I am frustrated that things are built not to the standard of 20 years ago. Today, you chuck the whole thing – a waste. It is a throwaway society.

I have loved airplanes since I was little. I always **felt I was so different from family on the universe and life's creation**. So different from their ideas. I always felt different.

Age 16, I had a car accident. I swerved to miss a car that wasn't there. It turned out to be my car. It was my car I had swerved from. **A time lapse of 2 minutes** into the future. I saw what hadn't happened yet.

Age 17: military, Air Force. I worked in airplane radar systems. Then I **tracked a UFO**. It would go 1,000s of miles per hour and then make a **90-degree turn**. This was later verified by NORAD. **I believe in UFOs**. I saw the object land. Then a long pause, and I lost one day of my life. I don't remember anything!! It made my mind crazy. The more I think of it, the more **my mind goes round and round and round**. I don't tell people. I am trying to remember that period of time. I remember being on a knoll there and looking back to the object, but I don't remember moving from there. Then the next morning, I was in the barracks. The fact that I can't remember is so prominent.

Flying and skydiving scared me to death for many years, but I had to do it. I go for high adventure, danger. It doesn't ever seem like danger to me. It is being like a bird and flying.

My parachute malfunctioned and I almost died. It didn't open. Why didn't it work better? Below tree line, it opened. Everything stopped motion. CLICK, CLICK, CLICK. I left my body and watched from above. I knew I would die; everything comfortable and it was OK. The parachute opened very, very close to the ground. It was like a huge vacuum, and sucked me back into my body. It was life altering – I appreciate life.

But now, I seem to have lost appreciation for life. I am not fulfilled, as if life is over.

As if the adventure gone. I don't fly or sky dive so much. Raising children. The real world. **I had to grow up. I just wanted to stay Peter Pan!**

I am irritable. I was always **a loner.** I don't bother people; they don't bother me. I have lost the thrill. **No fun anymore.** I used to have too much fun.

I take care of the kids. I'm the housewife, a female role. I don't feel appreciated.

I have no control. Life is run by others, and I'm along for the ride, doing what has to be done.

Now I can't decide. When I fly, I always make decisions of life and death.

No mishaps. I'm like a captain of a ship with no ship. Good in a crisis, I keep my head. I don't make mistakes. I have to do it right.

Q: What do you want help with a remedy?

I don't know. I want to be happier; something is missing. I'm not sure what.

The parachute thing – I felt robbed. Death was imminent – no question. I handled it ok, and was brought back. **I will have to face it again some time.**

Q: Religion?

No. Jesus values, being hung on a cross, are in all of us and we all are that person.

Q: Work?

I always said I can do anything for a short period of time. **I never reached a goal.** I didn't make 1000 jumps, or didn't fly 10,000 hours.

I can **make computers work**. I am mechanical; I like to know what **makes things tick**.

Generalities: High cholesterol and lipids.

Desires: cookies, pies.

Aversion: sweets, chocolate, candy.

Night sweats.

Nose: sinus problems.

Worse with cold, better with heat.

Dream: Recurring dream but can't remember.

The worst thing is being a housewife 24/7. **You've gotta have a break; there is no time.** But I don't want anything to happen to them (children) while I watch them.

Rx: Krypton 30c

Follow-up 2 months later

From wife: After 2 weeks, he had a deep and unusual realisation in the middle of the night. He had to wake his wife to tell her.

He realized that though he is not from here (from this planet), and though where he came from was a much better place, it is right that he is here and that this is where he should be. Since then, he is much more emotional in general and more interactive with people. This has made his fear of the UFO incident worse, but he is more aware of it. As if before, he was in total denial, now, it is more of an acute fear. He has begun interacting very warmly with our adopted daughter's mother, which he needs for the court case, and they talk for a long time on the phone (very unusual for him). He has more joy for life, and has gone back to building airplanes, which he had loved but had given up on. He is less particular, and less censorious about everybody getting it perfectly right all the time. A massive change.

No further follow ups recorded.

Jeremy's comments

This is a remarkable case with a remarkable story. It covers many of the Krypton elements perfectly. Once again, we see the painful transition from Argon's Peter Pan to a responsible but miserable adult. The strict and responsible upbringing leads to the love of freedom and flying but culminates in being a full-time parent and losing the joy of life. Further aspects such as intellect overriding emotions, the love of computers and physics, Hawkins and the universe are all there, as are the glitches in time and the circular nature of time. This case has the common noble themes of perfectionism, love of truth and aversion to company.

Of course, the UFO story is the strange rare and peculiar aspect of this case. The susceptibility was always there, he believed he was from another planet. Perhaps they came to take him home.

As in the first case we see the ecological care leading to aversion for people who destroy the planet. Finally, when he is in the zone, flying or skydiving, he is truly a superman.

CASE 13.6 Organised scholar

Homoeopath: Jeremy Sherr, Israel

Male, age 67

Background
The patient is a scholar and accomplished artist with much general knowledge. **A logician.**

Loves reading, reads 8 hours a day, and has a vast library.

He studies history and botany, and often quotes other authors. He likes books with **spiritual richness.**

Consultation
"I am an intellectual and a **perfectionist, pedantic.** Everything is in order".

He tends to be **very cynical**, and likes to play **mind games.**

He has a very quick metabolism, and has a stool the first thing in the morning after coffee.

He likes alcohol, cannabis, and cigarettes. This "helps me to deal with the everyday reality".

He has anger, which he got from his grandfather. The anger is not logical.

He urinates frequently.

"I check with my doctor every 3 months, and look after myself".

"I am very stable. I took many drugs but never lose my mind, never needed help from outside. I am against help from the outside. I don't believe in psychology".

He had a heart bypass.

It is "strange that I am still alive. I went to extremes, had an idle youth. I thought I would live an intense and short life. I am living longer than what I thought I would. Now I am getting old, and physiology is becoming a burden".

"I live alone, and am **very friendly with myself. I prefer to have no windows**".

"I don't want to fight with myself. I live with myself 24/7".

"When I wake up, I start from the beginning, start afresh. **Every time I wake**, I **just start again.** If I wake at 4 am, no complaints, I just carry on reading my book".

"I live horizontally, always leaning because of an elbow bone growth".

"I dream I go into a place with a problem and **find a way out or wake myself**".

"I'm not interested in self-examination or in examining others. I don't dig."

"My life is beautiful. I am strong emotionally. Maybe as a I was kid offended, now not".

"My culture and background are German, hence a perfectionist and love of culture. I can make order out of any chaos. I read systems well. I can organise a new system by families and every other category. I keep a logbook on everything".

"I stamp and record every phone call and the contents of the phone call. I create a framework. That way, I can check who called and what they said. I'm very pedantic".

"Because I drink, I put people off. People are scared of me, but I don't mind. Women are scared of me because I drink".

"The only game I play is mind games [teasing and trapping people – JS], and this can offend people".

"I am a bit childish emotionally, but I don't mind into it.

I have no commitments.

I hate injustice. Theoretically, any theory that is fixed or rigid like a diamond, in peoples' hands is a rag. Like Marxism or communism. That makes me sad, people live by ideology. I see the disconnection in theory and practice.

I am **sad that there is no perfection.**

I have no complaints; I live in my means with what I have. **Time is on my side!"**

At age 9, he had headaches.

A few years ago, had **heart** pain, like a toothache of the heart. He had a heart murmur as a child.

He has poor hearing in his left ear.

"I eat only when hungry. I can forget to eat; I have no interest in food, but I cook well, functional cooking".

"I don't like cold damp weather".

He has aversion to the cold.

"I don't like people, but I am very **intuitive**. I am not good at music and maths, but am good in abstract thinking.

Rx: Krypton 30c

Follow-up 2 months later
"I liked it. I am more optimistic, more positive. I am moved ahead; I feel the remedy has done me good. I am healthier, more flexible".

"I had many new dreams. I am decoding them; [they are] helping me to find solutions".

Rx: Krypton 30C

Jeremy's comment
This case is more balanced than the previous ones. There are none of the work issues, but the sense is of a very strong and organised intellect that overrides the "childish emotion". His perfectionism, cynicism and mind games are illustrative of this. He "never loses his mind". Everything is logged and catalogued in an orderly way. Even his dreams are solved logically while he is dreaming. He feels his anger is not logical, and non-logical emotions are foreign to him. He does not like to dig or to unearth them. He uses his sharp intellect to tease others.

He prefers to be alone, hiding in books and intellectual pursuits. There is no need for windows or help from the outside. Yet deep below, standing in contradiction to the intellect, is a strong intuition, a primitive animal side.

Once again, we see the use of alcohol and drugs in this case.

Otherwise, it seems that "Time is on his side", in that he lives a kind of continuum, each day beginning afresh in the present, and he feels his life is beautiful. He lives happily with himself 24/7. He did not expect to live long, but seems to enjoy and make use of every minute.

After the remedy, his emotions begin to rise in dreams, and he decodes them.

In this case, we see the characteristic heart pathology again, as well as the Krypton aversion to cold, damp weather and heart pains.

CASE 13.7 Spiritual scientist

Homoeopath: Camilla Sherr, Tanzania

Female, age 50s

Consultation
I have been working all my life. **I always work.** I started **working at the age of 11, and haven't stopped since.** Even when I had my daughter, I never stopped. I didn't really want her. I didn't want to be a mum. I just wanted to work. **I love the academia. I'm a researcher and a Fulbright scholar.** There isn't anything I haven't done in the academic world.

My daughter was a twin. Her sister didn't survive; they were born at 24 weeks. I almost died and so did she. Her body was the size of my palm and you could see all the organs through her skin. My husband looked after her mostly. I was the breadwinner.

I'm a Reiki master and a Sheikh from my husband's religion. **I have no connection between my head and my heart.** I live in my head, not in my heart. I'm all head.

[This is the scientist that came to Camilla's mind during her Krypton proving.]

Rx: Krypton 200C

Follow-up one month later
I feel so fantastic! I feel like the old me. In 1998, both my parents and my best friend died within 6 months of each other. I think I've been

in shock since, but now I much feel better. A lot better. I'm happy, I FEEL happiness. I laugh. I hug people, I'm more physical. I want to hang out with people. **I'm sick of working**. I told someone at work "NO" for the first time. I don't want to work. I want to drink beer and see my friends; enough is enough!

For the first time, **my head feels connected to my body**. I am more connected to my female side and intuition. I want to do new things.

My relationship with my daughter has improved and I spend more time with her. I enjoy her more. I feel her more.

Observation: During a lecture of hers which we attended, she mentioned the **5th dimension five times**. No one knew what she was talking about, I don't think she did.

I want more of this remedy! It's the best thing that has happened to me!

CASE 13.8 Recycled OCD

Homoeopath: Jeremy Sherr, Tanzania

Male, age 15

Background
Remedies from previous homoeopaths include Silica, Plumbum, Carcinosin, Chamomilla. Not much change.

The main issue at the moment is anger at trifles. If someone does something slight or interrupts, it annoys him.

He recently suffered an eruption of infectious impetigo.

He has vertigo on bending or bowing, or vertigo with a faint feeling on standing suddenly. Random faint feelings.

Consultation
If I get angry, I go to my room and then complain to my mother. I don't express it to the offending person. I suppress my anger.

I feel tired and exhausted. I am anxious about the skin eruption (impetigo).

I have anxiety about my health in general, and anxiety about irreversible disease.

I have **not shed my baby teeth**; I have two rows of teeth.

I left school, could not fit into that environment. I have **obsessive compulsive** disorder.

I have a feeling of not being listened to, no one listens to me. I am annoyed when others finish my sentence for me, from being interrupted. When friends don't listen, I get annoyed. Everyone is always finishing my sentences. *[He repeats this several times.]* I am afraid of others finishing my sentences. It happens a lot because I live with adults, not being listened to. I waffle a lot; I don't like if they come to the wrong conclusion from what I say.

I had dream of skeletons as a child. I dreamt something about **top of the mountain and the bottom** which annoyed me. I dreamt of a big chasm behind me.

Q: OCD?

I've always been there. When I walk in the supermarket, I have to **retrace my steps**: I go in a circle the way I came to undo the circle. I must always **go back the way I came to undo the circle.** Any circle I make, I must go around again to make it beautiful and not ugly.

If I make a mistake writing, I will not rub it out; I must honour the mistake.

I have to pick up stones and rubbish in the road. I personify them. I am afraid to insult an object by leaving it on the road and favouring another object. If I pick up one stone or bits of rubbish from the road, I have to consider the other stones and get them too.

If something must be a certain way, I must do it like that. I must always undo things so as not to hurt anything, even a mistake in my book.

I can't kill a fly or mosquito, once I did, and I felt awful. I go right back to the original regret.

When I was small, I had earaches with pus.

A strange thing is when I cry, the **tears go back into** my ears.

I am perpetually hungry. I always desire more food.

I had recurring dreams of my sister hanging up clothes by a chasm and slope.

I **bend over** to suppress my anger.

I have a strange sensation where I **don't feel the sum of my parts.** I feel like an arm attached to a leg, attached to a torso. Like a collection of bits tied together.

Rx: Krypton 12c, once daily for a week

Follow up three weeks later
My impetigo was better the day I started the remedy. Before, it was getting worse and worse, but now it's gone.

While taking the remedy, I slept for the whole week.

I am still stressed, but not as bad. Instead of being angry, I just slept a lot.

When I forgot to take the remedy, I got angry. But when I took it, I was sleepy.

My vertigo is better! I am less tired.

My OCD is the same. Or actually maybe there was some change?

But I am definitely less angry, less anxious about people finishing my sentences.

Follow-up six months later
A month later, he took Krypton 30C and recently 200C, one dose.

Soon after taking the Krypton 200C, he became very upset, frantic that he wouldn't remember "little stupid things" that were "**slipping out of my mind** like a handful of sand which I am trying to carry to the end of the beach". He began to **repeat key words** so that he wouldn't forget. He was distraught and could hardly speak through his sobs – though repeating the words compulsively.

Since then, he is doing very well.

The sensation of not feeling the sum of my parts is gone. It came back recently but vanished again after the last dose of 200C.

I have more energy since repeating the remedy, am more able to do things.

Nothing bothers me right now, no problems or anger. My vertigo is totally gone.

I have less OCD. Perhaps I am not under so much stress, but I haven't been getting it. I'm not picking up things as much. I was able to decide that the thing on the ground was happy where it is and walk on.

I have no anger from being interrupted, at least I haven't noticed it.

I've had no water going back into my ears when crying.

I had a dream of being in the police force and governing magic by building stairs. I was making sure people didn't misuse magic.

On the whole, I'm improving nicely. I am much less bothered by anything, all is milder and more gentle.

From Mother: He is doing very well.

Rx: Krypton 200c in 6 weeks

Jeremy's comments
This young man is stuck in a cycle where he must recycle or preserve everything. He has to retrace his steps so as not to break the circle. He recycles stones and rubbish from the road. He cannot erase a mistake. His biggest fear is that the cycle of his talk will be interrupted and of irreversible disease. His tears are recycled through his ears. His baby teeth are preserved.

It seems that the root of this need to preserve and recycle is a fear of things being lost forever: the stone in the street, the baby teeth, the mistakes in writing. Like Krypton, he has a dis-membered sensation. Perhaps the fear is that it may all fall down the big chasm of his dreams and vanish forever. Ultimately this chasm is the hole in the centre of his being where his body bits are joined together but do not form one unit, much like the skeleton in his childhood dreams. Like Krypton, he is dismembered. The fear is to lose the continuum.

One of the most instructive symptoms of this case is the dream of being part of the police that prohibit the magic, the Krypton-recycled brain controlling the Argon child.

CASE 13.9 Asperger syndrome

Homoeopaths: Camilla and Jeremy Sherr, UK

Boy, age 3

Background
His speech is indistinct, and very difficult to understand what he says, especially in English. His French is much better.

Consultation
He does not respond to questions; two-way communication is difficult. You ask him if he's hungry and he'll reply: Piglet is pink. He

seems to be in his **own world** a lot, or in a fantasy world with Winnie the Pooh or the Moomins. He **gets stuck on things, the same video, the same book, same toys, the same music**. He only listens to a specific klezmer music CD, puts it on really loud, and dances wildly around the room. He also responds in the same way, like when picking him up from nursery he will always say, "I had lunch!" He focuses on one thing only, but very intensely; you can't break his concentration. It seems that he lacks interest in broader terms, in a variety of things. He's not open to learning new things. It feels as if he's **locked inside** and shuts off the outside. He has **started closing doors and the rubbish bin** again (this symptom went away with Neon last year), he can't pass by them without shutting them.

He is very mischievous and destructive. He can't stand not breaking his train tracks at least twice a day. He laughs at reprimands, and thinks it's hilariously funny if anyone tells him off. He hates going to nursery school, cries every day and clings to his mother. He moans and whines a lot, feigns being hurt, very dramatic; "Oh!!! My finger!" He wants it kissed even though there's nothing wrong with it. He is very contradictory: "I want to go home. No, I don't want to go home. I want to go home. No, I DON'T want to go home. I wanna go hooooooooooome!". This happens many times a day. Just wants to watch TV all day.

He **repeats things**. He says, "Let's go in the car ... car ... car ... ar". He wants **to fly**, and is always saying, "I want to fly, high in the air". His favourite game is leaping down from the table or stairs, expecting someone to catch him.

Rx: Krypton 200c

Follow-up
The first week after the remedy, nothing happened; if anything, he was worse. And then suddenly, just like that, he felt normal. He started to respond in a completely different way. He would engage and answer back. When asked what his drawing was, instead of ignoring the question, he said it was an elephant. He started to be much less interested in TV. TV used to be his first question in the morning. Now he can go all day without mentioning TV at all. He has stopped whinging and whining. He's much happier. He had terrible night terrors about a week after the remedy, where he woke up and

thought things were crawling on his legs, trying to catch his toes. He was hallucinating, seeing things, and was in a complete state of fear and panic. It was like delusions but without the fever. He has had a few of these episodes in the past, when he was a baby. This time, it lasted from 12 at night to 4 am; and the next day he was better than ever. Like a complete transformation: happy, creative, he got that twinkle back in his eyes. He is now quite happy to try different things, parents have changed the music from klezmer to Tchaikovsky, and he's okay with that. His appetite is much improved, and he likes bananas again. (He used to love them and then went completely off them in the last 4 months.) He is much less clingy with mother; he likes his dad again, and will go happily with the babysitter. School mornings are easier. He doesn't fake being hurt anymore. He had one major episode of contradiction with self. After that, it was hardly there. He had the same train track from Friday till Monday without destroying it, which is a record! All the worries parents had simply vanished. He seems like a normal little boy, who instigates conversation, is curious and fun and seems to be relating better to other children as well. He is more interested in their company than before.

CASE 13.10 Down syndrome

Homoeopath: Jeremy Sherr, UK

Male, age 19

Background
The patient has been receiving Homoeopathy since the age of five. He has Down's Syndrome and suffers from a lot of ear infections, coughs and colds. He's had a number of remedies over the years, including Calcarea phos, Phosphorus, Nitric acid, Stramonium, Tuberculinum, Sulphur, Nuxvomica, Rad brom, Arsenicum, Carcinosin, China, Anacardium, Thuja, mostly with good effects.

Consultation
In October 1998, he came presenting symptoms of hair loss in patches and fungal toenails. He eats quickly and relates everything in his life to films he has seen, especially **"Groundhog Day"** (he loves

the idea of reliving the same day over and over again), 'Ghost' and 'Ghostbusters'. He is especially fond of movies involving **beheadings**.

He tends to talk to himself, and is **obsessive about time and routine**. He is heavily attracted to the paranormal, ghosts in particular. He says he wants to "save the worlds and **be a hero**".

While his intellect is good – **he loves reading encyclopedias** – his social skills are poor.

"He's really into the French revolution and republics. He's still keen to be a hero and an icon, that is, to be someone who is loved and admired by everyone".

Everything must go to plan, he has a very **fixed routine**.

Rx: Krypton 200C

Follow-up, 3 months later
Since taking the remedy, the patient's mother has noticed profound changes. He is much more patient, especially when things don't go according to plan. His communication is better, he talks more and is more able to express himself in a subtle way. He is **less obsessed with time**.

"He's obsessed with gases! Methane, butane ... He says he can feel it coming out when he breaks wind and talks about animals farting." However, he seems to be burping less.

His improvement continues.

CASE 13.11 Superman

Homoeopath: Doug Brown, USA

Male, age 40

Background
The patient, a married man and father of three, is jovial with hints of tension underneath, slightly formal, and eager to please me. At every visit he is unusually courteous and asks me if there is anything he can do to help me during my visit to his town. He says he wants to be my "best possible patient".

Initial Consultation, 2001

I have pain in my stomach, it's been diagnosed as duodenal inflammation by a gastroenterologist. I take Zantac (Ranitidine, an H2 histamine receptor antagonist). In the past, I responded very well to Arsenicum-album, 30C, once a week.

I had a stable youth. I lived in the same house my entire life. I was the oldest child in the family; I had three younger sisters. I did really well in school, through age 12. I graduated 5th in my high school class of 600 students.

I didn't go to college because I didn't have a plan, a major subject. I apprenticed with an uncle here in town. But there was not a lot of building. The economy wasn't growing. I moved around the country, going wherever there was work.

[Continues to tell a chronological story about the events of his life, meeting his wife, getting married, etc.]

I'm one of the luckiest guys you'll ever know. I'm blessed by my family arrangement!

I grew up without a television. I've been an avid reader. TV and movies affect me quite a lot. I wouldn't want to watch a horror flick. I tend towards **perfectionism**. I was a perfectionist in picking out my wife.

What troubles you?

Family troubles of my sister. Untimely deaths. I grew up in a close family. Some family members drifted to a different faith. I ask myself, what can I do to make the situation better?

What has been your most difficult experience?

The passing away of my aunt. I was pretty close to her.

What do you think is behind your stomach pain?

Little things in life stack up. I'm not smiling enough. I'm not paying enough attention to nutritionally balanced meals. I focus too much on my career and investments instead of my family, more on my career rather than my emotional well-being.

I resist change. I get **stuck in my routine**, my original plan. I'm contrarian. When someone says "I can't do it", I decide I *will* do it. Prove that it can be done (describes wallpapering a ceiling).

I had a dream where I'm in a **rocket ship**. It's shaped like a go-cart. My intention is to **fly into space**, though I'm sitting horizontally. I'm trying to familiarize myself with the controls. But it's not too important, because I'm the co-pilot, sitting in the second seat. A crowd around me, some say: "You know, it will make it to the moon and back. It's already been to Mars and back". Then I realized my wife was the pilot, and that she had been to Mars and back. I had been apprehensive because the rocket didn't look substantial.

Consultations between 2002 and 2011

Homoeopath: The patient was given many Kali salts, Causticum, Cobaltum, Zincum, Helium, Xenon, Syphilinum, Staphysagria, Palladium, Technetium, Cadmium-sulphuricum.

Patient:

I become totally self-absorbed. There is less recognition of others' strengths, with the power of teamwork. For example, building a house. If I say I can build you a house with no helpers, that gives a foundation for self-confidence. But if it takes three years to do it, the worth is not really there. When I hung the wallpaper on the ceiling, I employed techniques the others hadn't thought of to hold the paper up. **Gravity is working against you.** It would have been nice to have 8–10 people to hold up the paper while I worked. I stapled the paper with cardboard strips. The downside is that it's **lonely, alienating.** You **lose your ability to connect with others.** Consider Adam without Eve. You lose your sense of purpose. Why would you try to do something of value and worth? Who are you building it for?

I've reached the end of my comfort zone, and it's very turbulent. I'm looking for a breakthrough. I bounce up against a self-imposed ceiling, I need to break through an obstacle. I look for direction, guidance from my symptoms. I need a breakthrough to a higher level of health. It's like an aircraft getting ready to break the sound barrier, the buffeting of the plane. I'm seeing the **colour green.**

Joy from light and sound. It's a higher spot. A **mountaintop.** You can see clearly all around. One gets there not by working for it, but rather by receiving it. You open up oneself to what's beyond self. You get yourself out of the picture to see the beauty of larger creation. There's a **connection to a higher plane.**

I have **repetitive task-oriented dreams,** wishing I didn't have to do it again, that I could get something accomplished.

A dream of a very volatile, dishonest judge. Of people with evil intentions plotting a way to extort the town's citizens by threatening to blow up the dam and flood the city.

A dream of a lady whose **head was not connected to her body, a talking head.**

A dream of being arrested for having a small handgun. The officer was very jovial and nice.

A dream of **invincibility**. I have a magic hammer in my hand. Every project I take on is a total success. It's a wild west heroic feeling. I'm completely surrounded by bad guys. They can't touch me. You can take your time and bring them to justice.

I'm unwilling to accept change, e.g., my daughter driving, a new career, new roles for myself. I drag my feet through change. I'm **not the type of person to be spontaneous.** The hardest is moving from one job to another. I was stuck in transition when I was fired from one job. It was a management job at a lumber company. I put 110% of myself into that job. **I worked harder and smarter**, to do my best. When they said they wanted to let me go, I felt misunderstood, mistreated. I was offered my previous job, but I didn't want to go backwards, so I declined. I had future plans. I **was stuck in a transition**.

I fear being alone, vulnerable. I fear being unrecognized. Your individual needs are unrecognized, leaving you vulnerable. It's like being faced with an opposing force that's much stronger, without seeing a countervailing force. It seems insurmountable. Recognized means on the level of royalty. **I feel like a prince or a king.** Otherwise, I feel like a commoner. Not degraded, but not up where I like to be, on **a higher plane**. If once a month, you had the feeling of being like a king, the other days you could arrange your life so that it was an acceptable routine. But I would want to improve that to twice a month, and so on. On balance, I wouldn't want to think I was a king all day, when it wasn't true. It's deceiving yourself. Rose-colored glasses. A false feeling of I'm a king when I'm not. No one giving me individual attention. But still feeling **on top of the world.**

Trying to buy up the whole town. **I can do ten times more on my own.** I didn't need that job any way, playing the lone ranger. I can do it all by myself.

I have unreasonable expectations of myself. To be **"super"**. To have more happy moments. I wear rose-colored glasses. I have no regrets if I did my best. I recognize I'm a regular guy. **I'm not Superman.**

"Super" means I can accomplish everything by myself. It means I can go out in front, without risk to myself. I can take the heat for my family and friends.

If you could **look down on the whole world from the space shuttle**, it's that kind of perspective. That's the magnitude.

An email from the patient's wife describing a crisis: "Plans for family time didn't go as the patient planned. He had stopped eating "because it wasn't a priority"; he fainted, vomited."

Patient said he "was feeling so low, he was feeling sorry about having children".

Physical: involuntary hiccoughs, belching (**"It's a gas"**). Choking to an extreme extent, vomiting. "It is like a light switch on and off. When the switch is 'on', the food won't go down. Nutrients pass through too quickly to gain value." He has anemia, epistaxis, sinus congestion.

He has pain in his lower back, worse with inactivity, better with working. "My joints are not well oiled. My knees and elbows talking to me."

He feels weakness, is short of breath climbing stairs, has sore muscles, and a violence of symptoms.

I have back pain, so I took aspirin. Now I have stomach pain, worse at night, worse lying down.

I feel unworthy. It's a reflex to deflect praise. I have more success when working on behalf of someone else than when I work for myself.

I avoid conflict. Is there anyone more cheerful than me? A potential weak spot. I internalize negative emotions. I deflect praise.

If I didn't, I would fear a false advancement of self, setting up an environment of repeating success. A celebration of success, of taking praise.

If I was on stage and the presentation was successful, I think I could let the applause flow into me. But if I walked off the stage, and the audience member said "Great performance", I would say "Thank you", but that would be to deflect it away from myself.

Rx: Krypton 200C
[Following this remedy, the Homoeopath did not hear from the patient for 2½ years, a very unusual silence.]

Consultation, April, 2014
The last remedy cured me. I was feeling great until last month.

For the past two years, I didn't take any sick time. I'm cheerful and positive. I've been getting lots of work accomplished. I've been active, agile, and have good balance. I can walk a long way. I'm productive. I'm in control. I'm happier working with my hands.

In November, my employment contract ended. It was an opportunity to start my own business as a general contractor. But with the physical work, the heavy lifting, I found myself clenching my jaw, straining.

What was it like for you, starting your own business?

Contrary to what I expected, I never felt like competing. But the timing made sense. It's a step out beyond my comfort zone.

Dreams?

Dreams are **disjointed**. Faces I recognize, or don't recognize. Particular arrangements of chess pieces on the board. Feeling of surprise, unreality, things being out of place.

Chess?

It's about strategy; I'm drawn to different formations. I would like to win without capturing a lot of your pieces. That way it's a quick win, and I can relax. It's about control, being able to manage the game.

Rx: Krypton, 1M

Consultation, August, 2014

From patient's wife: Our relationship is better than ever.

Patient: Everything got a little worse for a few days, then better. My metabolism is quite fast. I do better if I eat, drink regularly. Otherwise I get bloated, have regurgitation, choking, and nausea.

I get some fear-based emotions when eating in a social environment, with friends, or family. Maybe it's a fear of failure, not exactly.

My sleep is good; my jaw pain is completely gone. I no longer get Charlie horses. I'm much better.

CASE 13.12 Spinning in a synapse

Homoeopath: Denise Straiges, USA

Male age 60s
I have a failing mind. It's been going on for a long time. Short-term memory – losing things.

I'm extremely high functioning so I'm aware of some very clear changes.

There's no correlation to stress or to drinking.

It's a **spinning in a synapse somewhere.**

Never been good with names now can't drum them up at all …

Handwriting has degenerated … my ability to write is significantly compromised.

Six years ago I moved out from where I was living with my wife.

We had been involved for 26 years, 13 years ago today we married. We're still married. She's the most stuck person I've ever known.

Been getting some psych help since 1991. At some point, a mention of killing one's self. The cause was my relationship. There are no drugs to change that.

Moved into my studio for a week. The relationship just trailed off after that. No fireworks. A very **private person.**

Work in archival conservation; I am **very precise** everything that I do. I **work a lot.**

Precise? Not a perfectionist … Not neat, not clean but overwhelmed for most of adult life. I have a ton of half-finished projects. If I finish one thing, the space is immediately filled with other things.

Fearful because of what's happening in my mind. Amped up because I'm becoming involved with a woman half my age.

My life is about **cycles and circles** of old projects. I do a project and then I have to write about it.

My mind works faster than my body … for example, if I write a 4-letter word, the first 3 letters are ok then the **4th letter becomes the first letter of the next word.**

Did neuro testing, MRI, 4 hours of quizzing. It's all decay and decline …

I got on a train this week going in the wrong direction because I **thought I was already at the place I was going.**

Recurrent sinus infections with yellow/green discharge and constant congestion. Had a lot of antibiotics.

Premature ejaculation since I could ejaculate.

I have the same problem with archery ... release too soon after fully drawing the bow. I don't hold it long enough. Everything goes too quickly.

Emotionally tight. **Keep a distance from people and myself.**

I've got many inventions ... **a problem-solving mentality.**

My life is paved with half-done, undone projects ... as soon as something is done I'm just on to the next thing. **It's cycling ... doing the same thing again and again ... it's a cycle of endless projects** ... once I see the end I lose interest. Guided by an intuitive process. I'm open to more projects than I can accomplish in one lifetime. Deeply unsettling ... More things come to me in a given day than I can respond to. On to the next thing. **Cycles of repetition ...**

I was raised to be a leader. Which is good because then I don't have a boss.

I want to be **more in my body than in my head.**

How can anyone function in a world with so much information?

Crave sweets, **dark chocolate.** Temperature is even, not much sweat.

Greatest pleasure is biking.

Responded well to Medorrhinum (in various potencies) for 2 years, during which time his chronic sinusitis resolved and memory improved. No change to the handwriting but he described himself as "moving forward." I didn't see him for about a year, after which he returned with a relapse of symptoms and I finally realized it was a Krypton case – which in hindsight seems so obvious with his fixation on numbers, time, and the endless cycles!

Relapse

Mind has deteriorated significantly; manifested into dementia. Can't remember words, unable to spell. Clumsy, off balance. Extensive typos. Using wrong words. Leaving stove on ... Putting salt in the fridge and milk in the cabinet. Can't tie a knot. Nothing is fluid. Sometimes when I stand I tip over.

I work at things but don't finish until the last minute. And then have to start something else. There's never enough time. **Time is the commodity that is most valuable to me.** I knew since my early 20s the importance of a **spiritual life, a meditation practice.**

So many things I want to do in any given minute. Goal in life to get everything done ... then would have a lifetime of projects planned in a half day. There are layers and layers in every second. I manage to be doing something in every second. I'm always thinking about time. For at least 25 years I have been unwilling to make plans on Saturday nights – that was for my own work – before the week starts over again. Ideas are like Niagara Falls. I used to suppress my urges so that I wouldn't have too many ideas.

My legs tingle. I think of it as hesitation about moving forward.

In my personal work there was never a message in anything I made. It's more about creating experience. **About being in the moment. About being present.**

Too many projects to do and any given one would have too many parts in it.

I'm **not in sync with time**. I have never been.

I'm very aware of the difference between having a cup of tea and just drinking the tea. I only do that about 3 times a year. It's hard for me because there are so many things I want to do – but at some level I cannot fully do it. I get up and think, I'm glad I've done that. It's over. **Now I do it again.**

Dreamed of people working out problems. The struggles of **being awake or being alive.**

Rx: Krypton 200C/1M

*First follow up showed significant physical improvement – no longer dropping things or tipping over. Improvements in speech but not as much in writing. Speaks mostly of his practices in archery and **Tibetan Buddhism** … impermanence.*

Increase to 1M potency, diluted for frequent repetition, was the key to unlock the Krypton mystery for this client after which he made consistent improvements in memory, cognition, coordination and capacity to "be" in the present moment. After parting company with the younger woman with whom he had been involved, he began to see himself "as a part of something bigger" and spoke of his emotional vulnerability and the openness of his heart.

At the time of this case submission, it's been six years since Krypton did its work, and the client thus far appears to have turned around from his descent into dementia.

Jeremy's comments
Great case from Denise. The main point is rushing forward into the cycles of time as opposed to being in the here and now. Spinning in his head, and out of touch with the body. All the other relevant points in bold.

CASE 13.13 Sun and moon

Homoeopath: Jeremy Sherr, Israel

Female, age 29

Background
She has been treated by me and others for over several years, with some improvement but nothing dramatic. She received Cygnus cygnus, Neptunium muriaticum, Agaricus, Nat muriaticum, Lycopodium, Platina and Ignatia.

The following is a compilation of symptoms from several consolations.

Her main complaint is a constant **pressure in her forehead** and around her eyes. She feels "**stuck**" in her abdomen. She is overweight through **sedentary work**, though she eats little. She has a very **strong desire for chocolate**. She suffers from poor sleep and clenches her jaw in sleep.

Her depression is much worse in winter, a deep sadness. She becomes suicidal.

Multiple consultations
When I feel good, I am like fire, high. When I am **enthusiastic, I fly high**; but then in a minute, I am on the verge of a narrow void. I feel that I will **fall in**. It is difficult to **remember that there is a God**; I can hardly pull myself out. I'm on the **verge of a void**.

I am sad about myself, the world. I have lots of self-judgement. The sadness comes from a lack of perfection, a **lack of wholeness, I am not fulfilling myself. Life is a burden.**

I was raped by my brother when I was a teenager. It all goes back to there. I could never tell anyone. My parents were not there for me. Then I was raped again in my twenties. **I am tired of life**, I just want to die. I feel **miserable**. But I am scared of **reincarnation,** so I don't kill myself. I just want a **rest from life,** to be loved by myself. I always struggle to prove myself to the world. I have lots of anger and suppressed anger.

I have a fear of heights. I'm afraid of what hides in the dark.

I have dreams of flying, very realistic.

My menses are painful.

I have a very strong **moon aggravation**. Everything is worse with the new moon and full moon.

I feel that my body has loads of energy, but it gets **stuck in my feet**. I feel I want to **cut off the soles of my feet** to let the energy out. This energy causes twitching in my pelvis. If I massage my feet, my whole-body trembles. All this energy is stuck and can't get out. It has something to do with the sexual trauma. I clench my jaw and grind my teeth. I have to keep myself under control, hold myself together so I don't collapse.

I prescribed Platina and Ignatia, there was some improvement and some new aspects of the case developed.

I am busy all the time, constantly busy.

So **much to do, I have no time**, I am tired and stressed. I want a **rest from life.** I am impatient with a short fuse. I have difficult concentration. My menses are painful.

I have begun studying **maths.** I feel that the **secrets of the universe** are coming to me in my dreams, in a **mathematical form.**

Rx Krypton 30C

Follow-up, two months later
I am so much better!!

I am flying with my feet on the ground. It is amazing!

I am doing wonderful things, I feel in the **present, here and now.** I look better, I feel better, I am happy!

I have had many colds recently, but it feels OK.

I kicked out my boyfriends; I am much happier. I have no more guilt. It feels great.

I am full and balanced; I have more self-knowledge. I am breathing properly, and I am centred.

All my physical symptoms are better. My **feet are not cut off,** my menses is pain free, the headache and pressure in my forehead are gone.

Rx: Krypton, 30C to take when needed, only if she relapses for over a week

Follow-up, six months later
I have been incredibly happy and healthy, happier than ever before.

I feel whole and protected, as if the **universe is sending me energy which flows through me**. All that I want is happening nicely, no symptoms, all is excellent.

Rx: Krypton 30C, when needed
This patient has not been seen since.

Jeremy's comments
Looking back on the case, the clues for Krypton were there all along. The sensation of the feet and abdomen blocking energy flow with a desire to cut the soles of feet off, the feeling of falling into a void, the fatigue from the burden of life, the depression, the difficulty in connecting to self and God, the fear of reincarnation, the typical noble gas desire for perfection and wholeness, the intense desire for chocolate, the pressure in the forehead, and the strong moon aggravation. As they say, vision is always 20:20 in hindsight.

Once I gave a couple of close, but not close enough remedies, the picture became clear. That is the secret of the second prescription. The busyness, the need for a rest from life, and the mathematical dreams were enough to indicate Krypton and justify her previous long-term treatment.

CASE 14.14 Asperger syndrome in 21-year-old male

Homoeopath: Camilla Sherr, Israel

Male, age 21

Background
Adult male diagnosed with Asperger syndrome, and suffering from OBS (Organic Brain Syndrome), displaying agitation, autistic stimming (self-stimulatory behaviour), flapping hands, clicking fingers.

Consultation

From patient's Mother:

I'm not sure that he understands a lot of the questions. It's difficult to know how much he actually understands. He wants explanations all the time, asking many questions. **Constant repeating**.

He keeps asking what do they (people) mean, what does this one mean with that? He is anxious, hates uncertainty, and hates things that don't go as planned.

Everything he does is just to have a plan to avoid the unknown. His brain is **constantly on schedules**. Once the plans are made known, he is much calmer. He suffers from anticipatory anxiety, is much worse with change.

He is unable to study, cannot concentrate, and has lots of **repetitive thoughts**. I often hear him repeating what someone else says. He also talks to himself.

He loves music, but it's always **the same song**.

He absolutely loves mayonnaise.

He likes to take responsibility about himself, and gets angry if reminded to do something. He is very friendly, prefers the company of regular children, and goes to youth movement meetings.

He **doesn't know what he knows**, and doesn't know how to bring it out. He doesn't know how to pull out appropriate information. If I ask, "What did you learn?" He responds, "I don't know". He is unaware of what he knows.

He fears gardening tools that make noise; balloons, because they can pop; sudden loud noises, but curiously he can listen to his music at full blast.

He doesn't like dogs.

His appetite is very good. Once he is outside the country, he is much more relaxed. In Italy, he eats, and walks around much more. He is better when he is pulled out of his surroundings.

He is up at night and sleeps during the day. As a child, he was hyperactive, but always slept [at night.

He has learning disabilities, verbally and visually. He is unable to follow what's going on in school, and he learns by action. You have to show him, step-by-step.

Planning is very important for him.

He gets on people's nerves, gets thrown out of groups, and doesn't understand the limits. He is obsessive, **can't stop his repetitive**

actions, and relentless in his actions. He can phone or text a person a hundred times in an hour.

He has a short fuse, takes his anger out on people, and then gets into trouble.

He's got his ups and downs, sometimes takes change well, other times he flips. Last week he got into very big trouble. He couldn't find his phone charger, and was cursing, and threatening. After it was found, he was very apologetic, and apologized profusely.

The school he's in wants him to leave; they can't deal with him. They say he needs to be hospitalized.

The school wants him to take drugs to be "balanced"; but we've tried it before, and it simply doesn't work for him. Those drugs don't help.

If he sees a change even one word, it's a whole different sentence to him. He sees the details.

Do you know that Asperger kids are used in the Israeli army to find **coding errors in complicated computer programs** and to spot changes in aerial photography?

He is very stubborn. He often says "Why am I so miserable" Why am I never happy? Why am I not enjoying life?"

He **remembers all the phone numbers. He likes the time to be exact**: half past or quarter to, and will fill in time to make it even.

As a child, he was hyperactive, and banged head against the wall.

He can imitate anyone, and imitates other people.

Regarding food: he likes meat, chicken for breakfast, and potatoes. He doesn't like rice. He likes fried, greasy things. Ice cream needs to be vanilla or light-coloured. He hates alcohol, and doesn't like sour, lemons, or pickles.

Time is very important to him. He learned the clock very early, and look at his watch all the time. He has never missed a bus or a train.

It is difficult for him to calculate or to be ready on time. **He was late for years.**

He talks to himself, and is always shifting position.

He has to be **left alone**, and needs to do his rituals.

The pregnancy was easy, the birth painless. He was a big baby. **His head was always a month bigger**. It was a completely painless birth. They asked me, "Do you realize you're giving birth?"

His speech very sophisticated, but I'm not convinced that he isn't forming sentences off by heart without really understanding what he's saying. He keeps asking, "What do they mean? What does this one mean with that?"

He does anxious planning. He is planning events 3 years from now. He feels the anxiety in his stomach.

He has no imagination. Anything abstract is very difficult for him to understand.

He has a circular brain. Since he was small, any circular motion was really attractive to him, like spinning. He would **spend hours in front of the washing machine watching it spin.** He could recite the cycle; the sounds the washing machine makes. He can spin a cushion on his finger.

He **can't understand linear, but he understands the calendar.**

He takes **circular walks**; he didn't like to turn back.

He does **not accept the fact that he is an adult.**

The year is over, and he is back New Year. He is obsessed with how time repeats itself.

His superpower is that if you give him any date – from the past, from the future, any date – he can immediately tell you which weekday it is.

It means that **he can travel in time. Picture Superman turning the planet around.**

Synthesis
This young man is stuck in a loop where time repeats itself.

Rx: Krypton 30 C, twice a week

Follow-up, one month later
His mood is better. His thoughts, obsessive, are happy by nature, and he has private jokes. He says, "I'm happy because I'm feeling much better". He has calm thoughts, and more calm thoughts.

He is more helpful at home. He keeps asking, "Do you need help?" and tells me, "You should compliment me."

He is quite active. He is definitely much happier, bothering people less, and texting less.

I asked him if he can master his obsession with phone and texting. "OF COURSE!!" he says with confidence.

He says "I feel changed. I have changed".

Follow-up, another month later
His repeating is better. His asking questions has changed. He now asks the questions in a way that is more acceptable to people. He seems to understand the answers better.

"Yes, I understand others better. I'm not so **wrapped around** myself anymore."

He has changed schools. He took it very well with very little anxiety.

He used to be very anxious about his bus not stopping at his stop. After the remedy, the situation resolved itself when he understood which bus to take.

Rx: Krypton 30C, continue as before

Follow-up, four months later
They have reduced the Risperdal, which was given for repetitive thoughts, from 4 pills a day to 1.

He has now realised that he is 21. It upsets him a lot. He keeps saying that he doesn't **want to grow up.**

Time has kicked in. A year doesn't just repeat itself. The endless cycle is now also linear. He is creating a spiral of life where time moves.

Rx: Argon 30C

Follow-up, two months after Argon
He is moving out on Tuesday, to an Asperger home, semi-independent living 30 km from home.

He was able to express himself very well in the interview! He seems to have grown up. He also says it himself, and people around him that he's matured. It has been one of the best summers we've had! Usually, summers are very difficult because of the unknown of it; no structure. The unknown has been a problem. This has improved. Also, his constant planning and writing messages, there is very little of it now.

He is much calmer.

We went to the school's end of the year party and were amazed how easily he has adjusted.

He tells "In general, I've been good. I have my moments, but all in all good."

When his mother goes, he now has no more anxiety. He solves his own problems.

His mother says, "I have to ask him less. He actually notices a need and responds to it. He does things, helps without having to be asked." He takes Argon weekly and uses rescue remedy.

He now says, "I want to be able to be independent, to manage my money, to live alone in Tel Aviv."

He was also able to express his goals.

He is better at using all the information that he has in a correct way. It's not so disconnected. He has no more repetitive thoughts.

He loves water; it makes him feel better. Even a shower helps. (Argon Neon?)

Jeremy's comments

Very nice and clear case, where we can see time and thinking stuck in circular movement. Linearity is impossible. The second prescription into Argon is also great to see, as if he is moving back up the periodic table, into the youthful Argon world which want to avoid the progression of time. Noble gases often follow each other well.

Conclusion from Krypton cases

The cases above all reflect and illuminate the proving nicely. It is really a joy when a proving is clinically confirmed and cures people, as well as allowing more insight into the remedy.

Two of the cases support the idea of Krypton or other noble gases occasionally suiting Down's syndrome, Asperger, or autism. However, it is plain to see that there is much more to this remedy.

What is common to many of the cases is an overactive intellect at the expense of emotions. There is little emotional content. Most of the cases have no big fears, no forsaken feeling, no anger or jealousy. In a couple of the cases, there is underlying fear or anger, but the intellect attempts to override these emotions.

All the aspects of the Krypton psyche are there – instinct and intuition, spirituality, rational and buried emotions – but they are not integrated with each other. It is as if the person is disconnected from themselves, dismembered; the head is cut off from the body and the torso is separated from the bottom half.

Feels as if upper torso is disconnected. Left and right across the upper part of my heart, and front and back at the lower.

Once the parts are cut off from each other, there is no energy flow between heaven and earth. This results in energy curving and looping, especially in the brain, like standing between two mirrors and having the image bounce back and forth. The third eyes turn inwards, thoughts repeat, the person becomes obsessive and pedantic, plays mind games, and remains stuck in a tedious loop. This loop is usually time-based: the daily repetition of work making one feel like a slave, a rat on a revolving treadmill with little enthusiasm. Responsibility and Monotony are the enemy. Creativity and mental challenge can send a current to buzz the Krypton light; but in the absence of these, the light goes out. This can often lead to drugs and drinking. The brain loop can also result in a stroke, the result of too much energy stuck in the head.

The intellectual loop manifests in repetitive thoughts that go nowhere and have little impact on the real world. Theoretical academia and research, mathematics, logic puzzles, cataloging phone calls, retracing one's path or collecting rubbish, all with a perfectionist streak. Time is an issue: it curves and loops, glitches or stagnates, and just occasionally bursts into a continuum. On the opposite side, when the Krypton patient may be a real hero when upright and connected to truth, energy flowing and karma shattering.

We can add South American shamanism to the spiritual Krypton affinity to Egypt and Tibet, all countries with pyramids, usually four-sided, and a mythological affinity for stars, UFOs and aliens. In two of the cases, we find the patients claiming to be from another planet, with an affinity to UFOs and a predilection for saving the earth. Superman anyone?

14

KRYPTON MM: ANALOGY, BIOLOGY, CRYPTOGRAPHY, COSMOLOGY

The following chapters expand into analogy, biology, history, religion, mythology, geometry, cryptography, philosophy, physics, and poetry. The study of higher concepts leads to a more profound understanding of Krypton and its use in difficult cases. One never knows where the all-important clue will come from, and it is good to train our minds to be perceptive on the highest levels.

This study will sharpen your senses as a homoeopath, because synthesising information and applying analogy and metaphor is the root of high-level homoeopathy. After all, simitars work by analogy.

Kryptonians

According to modern comic mythology, Kryptonians are an alien humanoid race of beings who originate on the planet Krypton. They are human in their structure and appearance, but their biology is far more advanced, and they can store and utilize their immense energy much more efficiently than Earth-based humans. While Kryptonians essentially exist in four dimensions, their senses are tuned to five dimensions, having developed superpowers such as super speed, heat vision, x-ray vision, and super breath.

Kryptonians, who are extremely advanced technologically, live isolated lives, only communicating electronically. Young children were known to be studying engineering even at the age of 5 years.[1]

Kryptonian[2] or Kryptonese, the fictional language of the fictional planet Krypton, first appeared as random squiggles in the Superman comics. Later, during the 1970s E. Nelson Bridwell evolved the squiggles into an alphabet of 118 letters. (Note: this is the number of elements on the periodic table.) In 2000 DC Comics created symbols for the English alphabet and issued a transliteration alphabet to decode writings in the comic books (Figure 14.1).

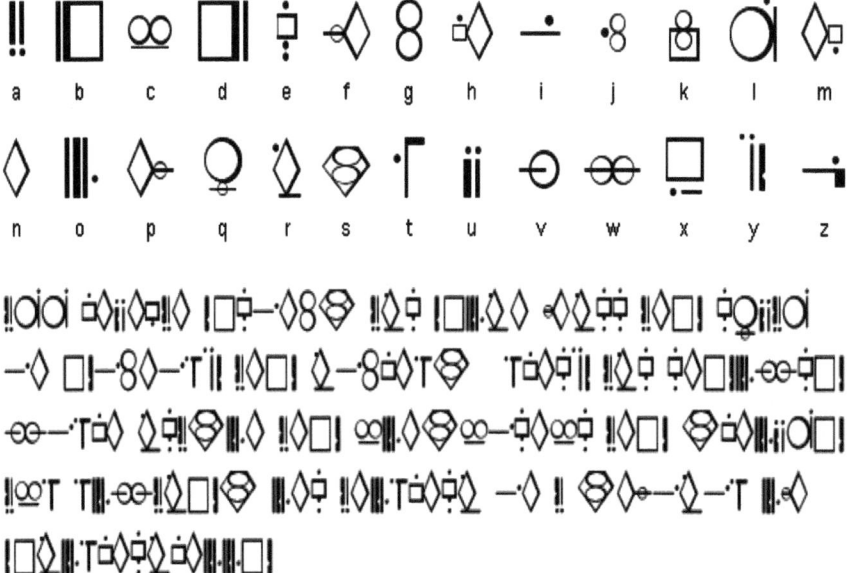

Figure 14.1 *Kryptonian alphabet above and Article 1 of the Universal Declaration of Human Rights*

Transliteration

(Article 1 of the Universal Declaration of Human Rights)

All human beings are born free and equal in dignity and rights. They are endowed with reason and conscience and should act towards one another in a spirit of brotherhood.[1]

Spaceland

Rudy Rucker, a science-fiction writer, mathematician and computer scientist, wrote *Spaceland,*[3] *a Novel of the Fourth Dimension* as a tribute to Edwin Abbott's *Flatland.*[4] While *Flatland* is a geometrical fantasy about a 2-dimensional being (A. Square) who receives a surprise visit from a higher-dimensional sphere, *Spaceland* describes the life of Joe Cube, a Silicon Valley executive who one day experiences new superpowers after a surprise visit from a fourth dimension being. For further description of *Flatland* please see my book *Neon.*[5]

Biology

In my *Helium, Neon* and *Argon* books I compared the evolution of noble gases to protein synthesis. Once a new cell is formed, it must create protein.

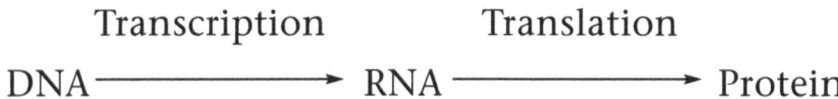

Transcription   Translation

DNA ————————→ RNA ————————→ Protein

Figure 14.2 DNA synthesising proteins

The instructions for protein production are transferred from DNA residing in the cell nucleus to the cell cytoplasm by means of RNA, where amino acids are constructed according to these directions. The whole process is known as DNA replication, transcription and translation (Figure 14.2).[6]

Helium is analogous to DNA replication (Figure 14.3), in which DNA duplicates itself during the early stages of mitosis, two strands becoming four. This is analogous to the four parts of the soul at the initial stage of incarnation. Neon corresponds to transcription in which the double helix unzips into two strands, one leading strand and one lagging strand. These strands are mirror images of each other. Each strand is then copied into a mirror image messenger RNA (mRNA). DNA has two strands arranged in a double helix, while mRNA consists of a single strand which is transported out of the nucleus to the cytoplasm. The remaining DNA then zips up

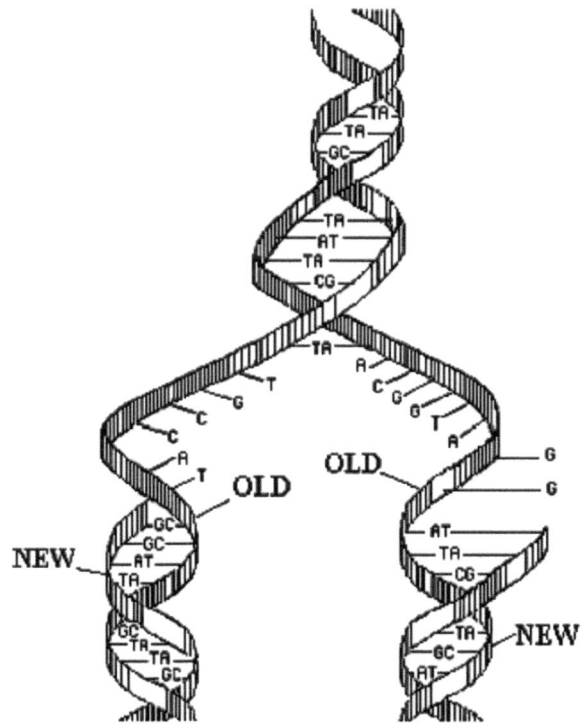

Figure 14.3 DNA splitting and replicating

behind it. Before entering the body, the four-part soul splits into two soul mates, each in a different body.

Argon corresponds to the stage in which mRNA migrates out of the nucleus and into the cytoplasm, passing through very narrow pores in the nuclear membrane. This passage is obstructed for other molecules, and so the process is analogous to the obstructed flow versus the free-flowing motion we find in Argon. The migration from nucleoplasm to cytoplasm can be compared to life's early passage from sea to land in Day Three, and to Abraham's migration to the promised land. Argon travels.

We arrive at Krypton. This stage corresponds to translation, the process of protein synthesis of **decoding** the sequence of an mRNA molecule to a sequence of amino acids. In mRNA, the instructions for building a polypeptide come in groups of three nucleotides called **codons**. The genetic **code** describes the relationship between the sequence of base pairs in a gene and the corresponding amino acid sequence that it **encodes**, which is basically **a mirror** image of the genetic sequence.

Transfer RNA serves as a link (or adaptor) between the messenger RNA (mRNA) **molecule** and the growing chain of amino acids that make up a protein. Each tRNA molecule recognises a specific, three base-pair mRNA code or **codon** (the DNA form of a codon is called a **triplet** and the sequence on the tRNA is called an **anticodon**) (Figure 14.4). Since there are three bases and four possible nucleotides, there can be up to 64 ($4 \times 4 \times 4$) possible tRNA molecules.[7]

Krypton codes. And decodes

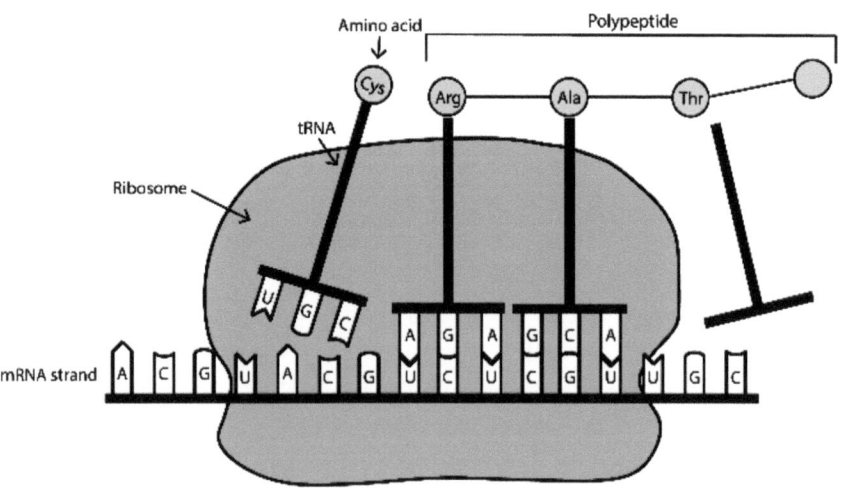

Figure 14.4 *mRNA forming mirror images with tRNA*

Alchemical stages, wedding of the gametes

In my previous books I discussed noble correspondences with the seven alchemical stages, and with the division of the cell. I was going to skip these in Krypton, as I thought the analogies were over. Then I noticed two curious things.

Argon had completed the process of meiosis, presenting the haploid cells of sperm and ova. In Krypton these two must unite in a new conception to form new life. This marriage begins in Argon, but its completion is in Krypton. Two haploid cells unite cells into a single diploid cell in the sexual conjunction of a zygote.

The fourth alchemical stage, conjunction, *represents the union of the masculine and feminine sides of our personalities into a new belief system or an intuitive state of consciousness.*[8] Conjunction leads to evolution of the spiritual self in its search for perfection when the learner can clearly discern the tasks to achieve lasting enlightenment. Conjunction takes place in the body at the level of the Heart Chakra and the body's sexual energies can be used for personal transformation.

So, I searched for weddings in Krypton, and discovered an aspect I had not previously noticed. This is how the game of analogy can help us gain new knowledge.

Dreamt I was in church to attend a wedding.

Dream we walked past a pool where a wedding was going on. The woman in the wedding dress was stepping into the pool, as if to be baptised.

Biblical and Cabalistic connotations[i]

Genesis

Earlier in this book I spoke of the relationship between the nobles, the dimensions, and the seven days of creation. I will now expand this discussion to portions of Genesis, the first book of the Bible, which is a blueprint of creation, and is built in fractal.[ii] To clarify, most of the ideas in this chapter are mine, not mainstream.

Genesis is divided into portions:

The first portion of Genesis
The first portion narrates the story of the seven days of creation, the second is about Noah, then the tower of Babel, then Abraham and on from there.

The following is a comparison of each portion to one of the days of creation, to the noble gases remedy pictures, and to the dimensions.

If we take the first portion as a whole, the one containing the story of the seven days, it is analogous to the First Day in which light and dark are created, as well as to Helium. The stories in this portion are one-dimensional; God and creation, light and dark, earth and water, sun and moon, non-sexual female and male with no shades of human complexity.

The second portion of Genesis
The second portion is about Noah. Yes, him with the Ark and the animals. This corresponds both to Neon and to the second day of creation; water, water everywhere. On Day Two of creation the waters divide into waters above and water below, but there is no earth. Later, in Noah's story, the great flood cometh, and again no earth. Water presents as a two-dimensional surface. Even Noah, a righteous person, is superficially presented as a two-dimensional character. The Bible only states that he was virtuous, in a naïve sort of way. He brings the animals into the ark two by two and survives the great flood. Even God presents as two-dimensional (from our flat point of view). At first, he is angry with Noah, later repenting and promising never to flood the earth again, a pledge he seals with a neon rainbow in the sky. The story ends with Noah getting drunk, reflecting the addictive side of Neon.

The third portion of Genesis
In the third portion, Noah has three sons, from whom all of humanity is born, and with them, the third period and third dimension of height begin to unfurl. In this portion, the people attempt to penetrate the height dimension by building the tower of Babel, which will reach the sky, but they fail and are scattered throughout the world, suffering an inability to communicate (Natrium) and confusion of identity (Alumina.) Alumina, clay, is flat and two-dimensional.

As clay earth it forms puddles, and if rolled into a 3-dimensional clay vessel it holds water, symbolising the separation of earth and water in the third day of creation. The world is still flat but poised for new growth.

Later in the **Third Day**, trees sprout into the third dimension. Three-dimensional space is created. As this dimension unravels, obstacles to movement are removed, resulting in free-flowing motion. Argon talks of easy, smooth travel.

The corresponding third portion of the Bible is literally called *Get going* – in Hebrew Leach lecha, לֶךְ-לְךָ - and tells of travel and crossing great rivers. Avram (later Avraham or Abraham) is told to walk 1500 km to the Promised

Land. Because he has crossed the great river (the Praat and Jordan) he is named a Hebrew – *he who has crossed the water*, like the many amphibians we find in the Argon proving. He then travels to Egypt and back again, where he freely wanders throughout the Land of Canaan and as far north as Damascus.

As height and trees develop, shadows grow, and personalities develop. This biblical portion is three-dimensional in its emotional complexity. Avram is a complex character, involved in two love triangles: the first is when his stunningly beautiful wife Saray is stolen by the Pharaoh. The second is with Saray's maid-servant Hagar. The rivalry between the two women concerns fertility and propagation, both prominent issues in Day Three, in which seed is created. Seed is mentioned several times in this portion.

Finally, in true Argon manner, Avram and Saray do not come of age or become fertile until their 90's, when they finally mature by becoming Abraham and Sarah. Their relationship with God also matures, extending beyond the simple concepts of good and bad into a mature set of covenants.

Once the third period is completed in Argon, the Bible moves into the fourth period and fourth dimension of measured time. Prior to this, there is a strange phenomenon concerning time, an eternal youth. People live to the ripe age of nine hundred and continue to have children at well over a hundred years old.

> *Adam had been living for a hundred and thirty years when he had a son like*
> *himself, after his image, and gave him the name of Seth:*
> *And after the birth of Seth, Adam went on living for eight hundred years, and had*
> *sons and daughters:*
> *And all the years of Adam's life were nine hundred and thirty: and he came to his*
> *end.*
> *And Seth was a hundred and five years old when he became the father of Enosh:*
> *And he went on living after the birth of Enosh for eight hundred and seven years,*
> *and had sons and daughters:*
> *And all the years of Seth's life were nine hundred and twelve: and he came to his*
> *end.*
>
> Genesis: Chapter 5[9]

Here follow several more examples of people childbearing at over 100 years old and living exceedingly long lives, until we reach the oldest person of all time.

> *And Methuselah was a hundred and eighty-seven years old when he became the*
> *father of Lamech:*
> *And after the birth of Lamech, Methuselah went on living for seven hundred and*
> *eighty-two years, and had sons and daughters:*

> *And all the years of Methuselah's life were nine hundred and sixty-nine: and he*
> *came to his end*
>
> Genesis: Chapter 5[9]

OK, this is weird. People having kids at 180 and living to over 900? No reasonable explanation given. Some scholars say these were symbolic ages, some say God was angry and shortened human lifespans. Perhaps the years were measured differently then, maybe the speed of earth's spin around the sun or on its own axis slowed down? Whatever the case, things are not what they used to be. Celestials' positions have changed.

343 degrees. The 17, 18, is not quite what we see now. It's what we used to see. Whatever this substance is it sees the heavens differently than what we see now, so the angle of the milky way and the big dipper is different to what we see now.[iii]

From our perspective we are moving from the third dimension into the fourth dimension, from the timelessness of Argon into the restricted, measured time of Krypton, and from there deathwards. Soon after the Biblical narrative above, lives begin to shorten. While Noah lives till 950, Abraham dies at the young age of 175, and Moses a mere 120 years,

Here is Genesis, Chapter 6:

> *And after a time, when men were increasing on the earth, and had daughters,*
> *The sons of God saw that the daughters of men were fair; and they took wives for*
> *themselves from those who were pleasing to them.*
> *And the Lord said, my spirit will not be in man forever, for he is only flesh; so, the*
> *days of his life will be a hundred and twenty years.*
> *There were men of great strength and size on the earth in those days; and after*
> *that, when the sons of God had connection with the daughters of men, they*
> *gave birth to children: these were the great men of old days, the men of great*
> *name.*
>
> Genesis: Chapter 6[10]

It appears that the change happens when the aliens landed: Sons of God, people of great strength and size, kryptonite supermen, or Titans. All definitely extra-terrestrials. And naturally they fancy the sweet, earth women. Who wouldn't? They have kids together, and the human lifespan drastically reduces. God brings in time cycles.

> *While the earth goes on, seed time and the getting in of the grain, cold and heat,*
> *summer and winter, day and night, will not come to an end.*
>
> Genesis: Chapter 8[11]

[iii] This is a proving symptom; I understand the 17/18 to be the difference between 343 and 360 degrees. Perhaps 18 relates to Argon. I don't know.

The aliens are here to stay, at least for a while. Three strange men, angels, extra-terrestrials, appear at Abraham's tent, and promise him a child from his ninety-year-old wife Sarah. Shortly after, two of them arrive at Sodom town. When the mob tries to lynch them, they blind them with a flash of light. Laser? Soon after, Sodom is decimated in something of a nuclear explosion.

The age of Krypton had arrived. Curved time space creates gravity, and it is gravity that pulls us to the grave.

Adam and Eve

Previously in the *Noble Gases* book series, we compared Helium to the androgenous Adam and Eve, a fourfold unisex existing in one body. Neon divides them into two sexes, and Argon finds them in the garden, just before eating from the Tree of Knowledge. Now that they have knowledge, they see each other's nakedness, compare and find that they are different, and cover up. God will not be pleased. Punishments follows, and we enter Krypton.

Man will have to **work hard** all his life, and Wo-man will suffer **labour** pains. The snake will **lose the use of his legs**. Humans lose immortality and are kicked out of the timeless, magical Argon Garden into the time-based world of work, taxes and death. Guarding the gateway (stargate) is an angel with a revolving sword, a mirror which reverses all images. Everything reverses in the krypton mirror, and this coded illusion will prevent us from finding the way back. When we see the gate to truth, we will not recognise it, but turn around and wander in the opposite direction, condemned to an everlasting, chronic search for the unattainable. And that is how our lives look today. If you want to find the way back through the mirror, remember this code crack:

The gateway to higher truth is through paradox.[iv]

Obadiah

Dreams of Obadiah, about Peter being ill. But it also spelt reptile and Copernicus and Galileo, Galilei and Galilee.

Obadiah is a little-known prophet with the shortest book in the Old Testament. His name means *He who **works** for God*, which is interesting in the context of the two types of work in Krypton: Timeless God Work and

---

[iv] (The original quote by John O'Donahue, was modified by me – after two beers!)

Tedious Human Time. In the book of Obadiah we see the themes of coming down from a lofty mountain, slip-sliding away.

Here is a portion of the book:[12]

> The pride of your heart has deceived you, you who live in the clefts of the rocks and make your home on the heights, you who say to yourself, 'Who can bring me down to the ground?' Though you soar like the eagle, and make your nest among the stars, from there I will bring you down.

The heart feels far away, difficult to reach. As if we are sliding helplessly down from the lofty mountain of love and there is nothing, we can do about it. This is scaring us. Song stuck in our heads 'Slip sliding away.'

Dream: I landed onto the highest place from somewhere in the universe to the highest mountain ... and I was descending ... descending towards the lower plains of existence

The righteous 36

Argon is element number 18, symbolising 'Chai' or 'life' in Hebrew. Krypton, the next noble gas, is element 36. According to Jewish tradition there are 36 righteous people living in the material world at any given time. The number 36 is pronounced as Lamed-Vav, which can be abbreviated to LAV or love. The Lamed Vav people live among us but will not be noticed because they are extremely humble. They are privileged to see the Divine Presence, and the world exists on their merit. Cabbalistic writings claim that these 36 righteous beings can cross the gateway back to eternal life.[13]

The 36 righteous ones are said to prophesise by means of a mirror. Like Alice in Wonderland, they can reverse restricted deathward time back to timeless truth by gazing through the mirror. They know how to pass through the angel's revolving sword at the gate of the Garden of Eden. This means they can transfer from the fourth period to the third period and beyond.

The number 36 in this context may have been taken from the astrological belief in 36 celestial decans, each of which rules ten days of the year and, thus, ten degrees of the constellations.

Cabbalistic geometry

Those who worship stars and star signs, rather than the one God, are considered 'curved' (עכו"ם), and not aligned with the straight line of the righteous. (kav ak'um and kav Yashar- curved line and straight line.)

72

In Cabbalah, God has 72 names, a number that comes up in the proving.[14]

2*36

References

1 Kryptonians. *DC Database*. Available online at http://tinyurl.com/yr8jdkm4 (accessed July 17, 2023).
2 The Languages of Krypton. *Kryptonian*. Available online at: www.kryptonian. info (accessed July 17, 2023).
3 Rucker R. *Good Reads – Spaceland*. Available online at: http://tinyurl.com/ 3s42r45w (accessed July 17, 2023).
4 Abbott E. *Flatland: A Romance of Many Dimensions* (1884). Available online at: http://tinyurl.com/475hp9yc (assessed January 20, 2024).
5 Sherr J. *Dynamic Materia Medica of the Noble Gases: Neon*. Glasgow: Saltire Books, 2016.
6 Miller C. Protein Synthesis. *Human Biology*. Available online at http://tinyurl. com/fzrcwe5d (accessed July 27, 2023).
7 Translation. *Biology Library*. Khan Academy. Available online at: http://tinyurl. com/tayvtxrc (accessed July 17, 2023).
8 de Giorgo L. 7 Stages of Alchemical Transformation. *Deep Trance Now*. Available online at: http://tinyurl.com/3fbskp54 (accessed July 17, 2023).
9 Genesis: Chapter 5. *Bible in Basic English*. Available online at: http://tinyurl.com/ mr2ankcw (accessed July 17, 2023).
10 Genesis: Chapter 6. *Bible in Basic English*. Available online at: http://tinyurl.com/ 364zvt4r (accessed July 17, 2023).
11 Genesis: Chapter 8. *Bible in Basic English*. Available online at: http://tinyurl.com/ mueu65pb (accessed July 17, 2023).
12 Obediah. *Bible Hub*, Available online at: https://biblehub.com/obadiah/1-3.htm (accessed July 17, 2023).
13 Lamed Vav Zaddikim. (Heb. 36, צַדִּיקִים ל"ו) *Jewish Virtual Library*. Available online at: http://tinyurl.com/2fbv8c3e (accessed July 17, 2023).
14 Daniel C. The number 72. *The Phoenix Enigma*. Available online at: https:// thephoenixenigma.com/72-2 (accessed July 17, 2023).

15

THEORETICAL KRYPTON CASES

The following are some theoretical Krypton cases, taken from people or symptoms in the proving or remedy symptoms. This is not a matter of pathology; Maybe these individuals would benefit from a Krypton remedy and maybe not, but their stories give a broad idea about possible aspects of the remedy. It is surprising how many contenders there are. Perhaps some of the Krypton people are such bright stars that they become famous. You will notice the constant battle between heart and mind, logic and nonsense, religion and rationality, all through the looking glass.

The following are by no means full resumes and biographies, just a collection of interesting facts that are related to the remedy, for your entertainment. The bold type indicates significant points.

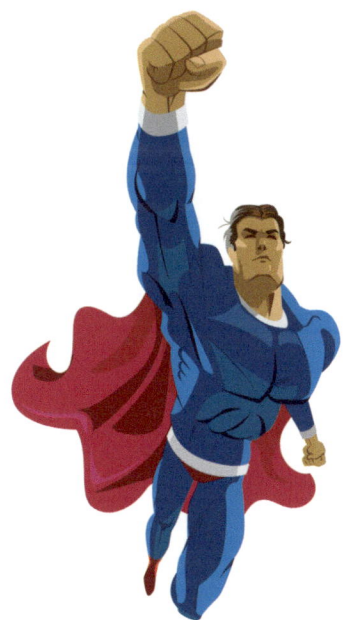

Superman (1938–Infinity)

Stars aren't measured by how long they burn ...
but by how brightly.

Superman was born on the fictional planet Krypton, which was disintegrating. To save their baby, his parents send him to Earth, where he acquired his superpowers, including flight, X-ray vision, unlimited strength, and a few more. Superman also **knows just about everything**. The noble hero dedicates himself to upholding "**Truth**, Justice and the American way." He **cannot lie**. Kryptonite, a green mineral originating from the planet Krypton, is the only substance that has the capability of neutralizing his superpowers.[1]

Figure 15.1 Superman

In the first movie, Superman **reverses time** by flying so fast around the Earth that it rotates in the opposite direction.

Christopher Reeves, who acted as Superman in four movies, was paralyzed from the head down in a horse-riding accident. He remained a **brain without a body** for the rest of his life.[2]

Another supervillain hero from DC comics is the Riddler, who Possesses a genius intellect and creates elaborate puzzles and nasty traps. The Riddler's **brilliance, neurosis, and lack of** empathy make him an incredibly dangerous foe. He cares very little about the lives of those he uses in his plots and sees them as disposable pawns in his **intellectual battle** against Batman.[3]

Leonardo da Vinci (1452–1519)

The noblest pleasure is the joy of understanding.

Leonardo da Vinci[4]

Truth was the only daughter of Time.

Leonardo da Vinci[5]

Leonardo da Vinci, a painter, scientist, draughtsman, engineer, sculptor, and architect, was one of the greatest geniuses in human history. He studied and kept prolific notebooks on anatomy, **astronomy**, biology,

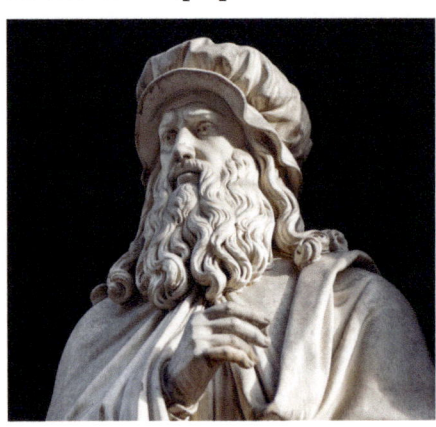

mathematics, physics, botany, geology, and **cartography**.

Leonardo researched the principles behind **light** and the flow of water, the growth of plants, and the stratification of rocks. His method was to draw and describe things by observing the surface before delving into the underlying structure. His notes were carefully documented and precise.

Among Leonardo's many inventions were the double hull, flying machines, a submarine, **a**

*Figure 15.2 Leonardo da Vinci * 1452–1519)*

calculator, an armoured fighting vehicle, and concentrated solar power **using mirrors**.[6]

In the context of Krypton, it is interesting that Leonardo loved **codes**. Historians and artists have discovered that many paintings by Leonardo contain optical illusions and hidden codes that cannot be seen with the naked eye, for example, a series of figures, letters and symbols in the eyes of the Mona Lisa, one of these being the number **72** (2*36).[7]

His notes were written in **mirror writing**, possibly to disguise the content. He became so adept at this technique he no longer needed a mirror to write in this way. He was ambidextrous, able to write with one hand and draw with the other at the same time.[8]

Likewise, Leonardo was fascinated by the **symmetry** of the human body and finding the place in which the soul dwells. He dissected many corpses, and these experiments resulted in one of his most famous drawings, the Vitruvian Man (Figure 15.3). The figure has **four arms** and **four legs**, depicting the union between man, geometry, and spirituality.[9]

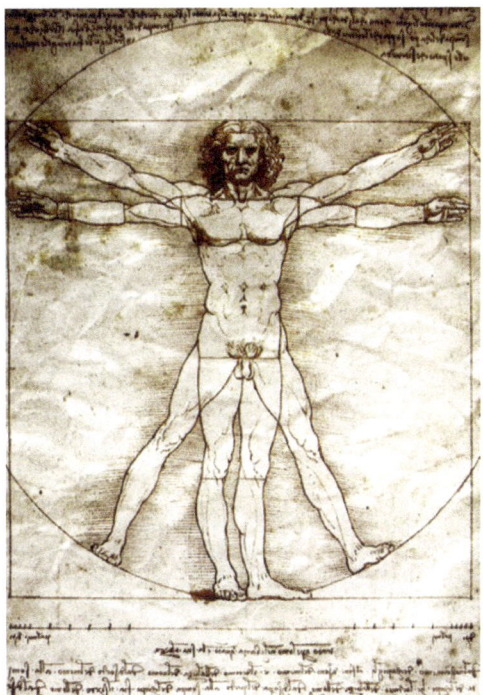

Leonardo utilised a special sleeping formula: he slept ¼ **of an hour every 4 hours**, meaning one and a half hours daily instead of eight (with a 75%-time savings in which he could be creative). He used this polyphase sleep for many years of his life without experiencing fatigue.[10]

Finally, the noble Leonardo was a vegetarian for humanitarian reasons. He would also buy caged birds in the market and release them.[11]

Figure 15.3 Vitruvian Man. (Leonardo da Vinci)

Nicolaus Copernicus (1473–1543)

To know that we know what we know, and to know that we do not know what we do not know, that is true knowledge.

Copernicus[12]

Of all things visible, the highest is the heaven of the fixed stars.

Copernicus[13]

Nicolaus Copernicus was a Polish astronomer and mathematician known as the father of modern astronomy. He was also a physician, economist,

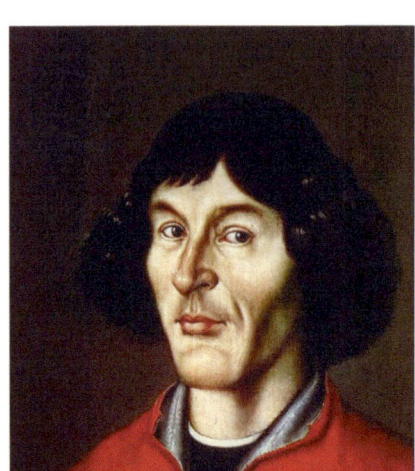

Figure 15.4 Nicolaus Copernicus (1473–1543)

translator, diplomat, Catholic canon and scholar of the classics and arts. He spoke Polish, German, Greek, Latin, Italian and Hebrew.[14]

After centuries of belief in the geocentric universe (in which the sun rotated around Earth), Copernicus suggested that the reverse was true. In his treatise '*On the Revolutions of the Celestial Spheres*', Copernicus presented a heliocentric model of the universe, in which the **Earth rotated around the sun**. Copernicus correctly suggested the order of the known planets away from the sun and estimated their orbital periods relatively accurately. He also postulated that the Earth turned daily on its axis and that gradual **shifts of this axis** accounted for the changing seasons.[15]

Lewis Carroll (1832–1898)

> It's no use going back to yesterday, because I was a different person then.
>
> Lewis Carroll[16]

> If everybody minded their own business, the world would go around a great deal faster than it does.
>
> Lewis Carroll[17]

> Alice: 'How long is forever?'
> White Rabbit: 'Sometimes, just one second.'
>
> Lewis Carroll[18]

Lewis Carroll[19,20] pseudonym of Charles Lutwidge Dodgson (1832–1898), was the author of *Alice's Adventures in Wonderland* and its sequel, *Through the Looking-Glass*. He was also a **logician, mathematician, photographer, and nonsense writer**.

One of his colleagues described Dodgson as '**austere, shy, precise, absorbed in mathematical reverie**', watchfully tenacious of his dignity, stiffly conservative in political, theological, social theory, **his life mapped out in squares** like Alice's landscape. In March 1856 he published a poem called **Solitude**.[21]

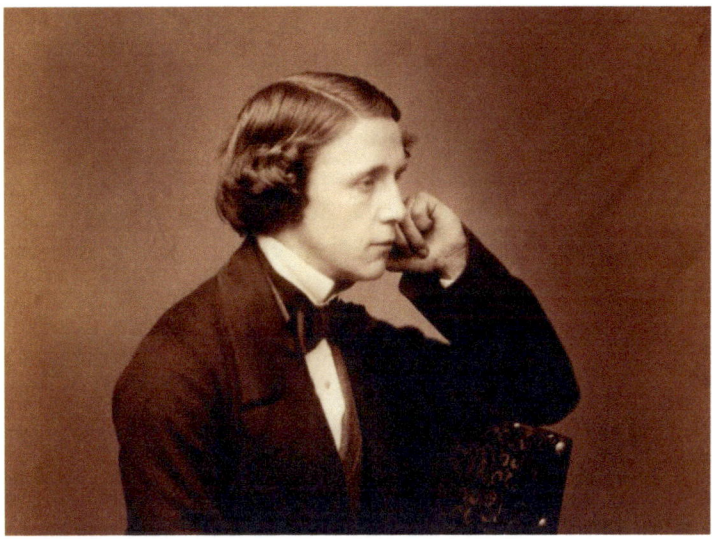

Figure 15.5 Lewis Carroll (1832–1898)

As a child young Charles began writing **riddles and puzzles**, in particu-lar **mirror writing**. He wrote a diary of 14 volumes, many of which had codes embedded in them. The name Lewis Carroll was a play on his real name, Charles Lutwidge, translated into Latin as. *Carolus Ludovicus*. He then translated it back into English as Carroll Lewis and reversed it to make Lewis Carroll.

His father, an Anglican minister and scholar, did a double first in math. Charles himself was a gifted professor of mathematics and wrote 11 books on linear algebra, geometry, and puzzle-making, including *Euclid and His Modern Rivals*. In a well-known article named *"What the Tortoise Said to Achilles"*, published in the philosophical journal *Mind*, Dodgson (Lewis) tells of the clever tortoise who challenges Achilles to a **battle of logic** which he wins by leading him into an argument of infinite regression.

Dodgson has many inventions to his name.[22] An early version of scrabble, a formula for finding the day of the week for any date (which some autistic children can do naturally); a device for notetaking in the dark, consisting of a **gridded card with sixteen squares** and a system of symbols; a device for helping a bedridden invalid to read from a book placed sideways; rules for calculating a win in betting; rules for dividing a number by various divisors; and at least two systems of **cryptography**. He popularized the 'doublet' a form of brainteaser still popular today, changing one word into another by altering one letter at a time, each successive change always resulting in a genuine word. For instance, CAT is transformed into DOG by the following steps: CAT, COT, DOT, DOG.

On own now, now own one, no own now, own one/won, we won?

Dodgson was an accomplished photographer, starting soon after photography was invented. At the time he had to develop the image from a plate immediately, which created a **mirror image**.

Carroll wrote many poems with acrostics. These are a poem, or series of lines in which certain letters, usually the first in each line, form a name, motto, or message when read in sequence. Through his looking glass, Carrol reversed logic into gobbledygook by penning several nonsense poems, including the classic *Jabberwocky*. Here is a section of his *The Walrus and the Carpenter*. There are several pointless interpretations of this, but personally I can see hints of the seven days of creation and in particular Day Four, which Dodgson would have been familiar as he was a deacon in the Church of England.

> The sun was shining on the sea,
> Shining with all his might:
> He did his very best to make
> The billows smooth and bright –
> And this was odd, because it was
> The middle of the night.
>
> The moon was shining sulkily,
> Because she thought the sun
> Had got no business to be there
> After the day was done –
> 'It's very rude of him,' she said,
> 'To come and spoil the fun.'
>
> [....]
>
> "If seven maids with seven mops
> Swept it for half a year,
> Do you suppose," the Walrus said,
> "That they could get it clear?"
> "I doubt it," said the Carpenter,
> And shed a bitter tear.
>
> "O Oysters, come and walk with us!"
> The Walrus did beseech.
> "A pleasant walk, a pleasant talk,
> Along the briny beach:
> We cannot do with more than four,
> To give a hand to each."

Lewis Carroll
Please see my poem *Wednesday*, p46.[23]

Isaac Newton (1643–1727)

Gravity explains the motions of the planets, but it cannot explain who sets the planets in motion.

Isaac Newton[24]

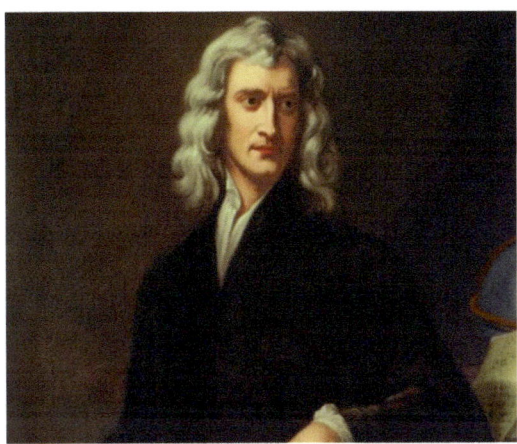

Figure 15.6 *Sir Isaac Newton ((1645–1747)*

In his *Philosophiae Naturalis Principia Mathematica*, Isaac Newton published theories about the laws of motion and gravity, the **celestial bodies, orbital dynamics** and tidal theory, all of which he backed up with **mathematics.**[25]   Though Newton is best known for his contributions to **physics, astronomy, maths, and calculus**, he also set the foundations for physical optics and built the first reflecting telescope. Newton was a student of **theology.**

Isaac Newton is widely regarded as being **autistic.** This is what his secretary had to say about him:

> I never knew him to take any recreation or pastime either in riding out to take the air, walking, bowling, or any other exercise whatever, thinking all hours lost that was not spent in his studies, to which he kept so close that he seldom left his chamber except at term time when he read in the schools as being Lucasianus Professor, where so few went to hear him, and fewer that understood him, that ofttimes he did in a manner, for want of hearers, read to the walls. [...] So intent, so serious upon his studies, that he eat very sparingly, nay, ofttimes he has forgot to eat at all, so that, going into his chamber, I have found his mess untouched, of which, when I have reminded him, he would reply – 'Have I?' and then making to the table, would eat a bit or two standing, for I cannot say I ever saw him sit at table by himself.[26]

Irritable Rabbi

Dreamt the rabbi was in a pale suit with three others, doing a Jewish ceremony. Was I to be the fourth?

The rabbi says it's okay if I have an H in my name. H and A are the same in mirror image.

The doorway was blocked so I had to go past the rabbi, who fortunately ignored me.

There was a conversation between Keppler, Newton, Einstein, and a very irritable Rabbi. They talked about gravity for the rest of the night.

It seems that a mathematical astronomical Rabbi appears in the proving. It took me some time to find him, but I think I have.

Rabbi Abraham Zacuto (1452–1515)

Rabbi Abraham Zacuto was born to a Jewish nobility family in Salamanca, kingdoms of León and Castile, Spain, where he acquired a thorough Jewish and secular education.[27]

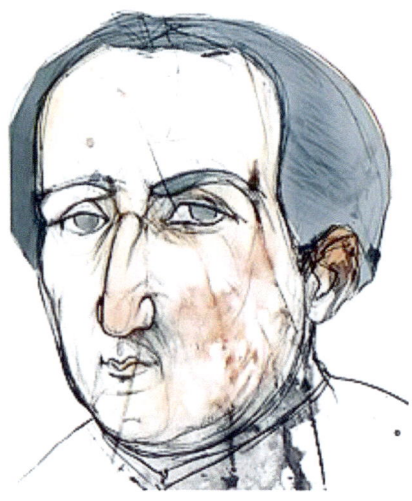

Figure 15.7 *Rabbi Abraham Zacuto (1452–1515)*

Zacuto soon became famous as an excellent **mathematician and astronomer**. He was awarded the chair of astronomy and mathematics at the *University* of Salamanca. His principal claim to fame is the great astronomical treatise *Ha-ḥibbur ha-gadol* (The Great Book), charting the positions of the Sun, Moon, and planets. His other astronomical work, called *Biur Luhoth*, written in excellent scholarly Hebrew, was translated into Latin, as *Almanac Perpetuum*, and immediately revolutionized **ocean navigation**. It was a great practical tool for the European discoverers who were about to explore the American continent and other far-flung areas. After this discovery, they were able to forge new sea routes into the unknown oceans instead of following the ancient routes along the coasts as had been done till then. This revolution in navigation changed the world map.

Astronomers from all over the world came to hear him lecture on mathematics and astronomy and sought his advice and opinion. Before setting on the voyage to India in 1496, Vasco da Gama and his crew underwent a thorough preparation by Zacuto, in addition to learning to use the new instruments which he had developed for their trip.

Irritable? This personality trait may have been depicted in a well-known 1572 epic poem, where a Zacuto-like character chastises da Gama for seeking fame and warns of risks ahead.[28] Figure 15.8 shows a 1936 painting by the English artist John Henry Amshewitz of Vasco da Gama leaving

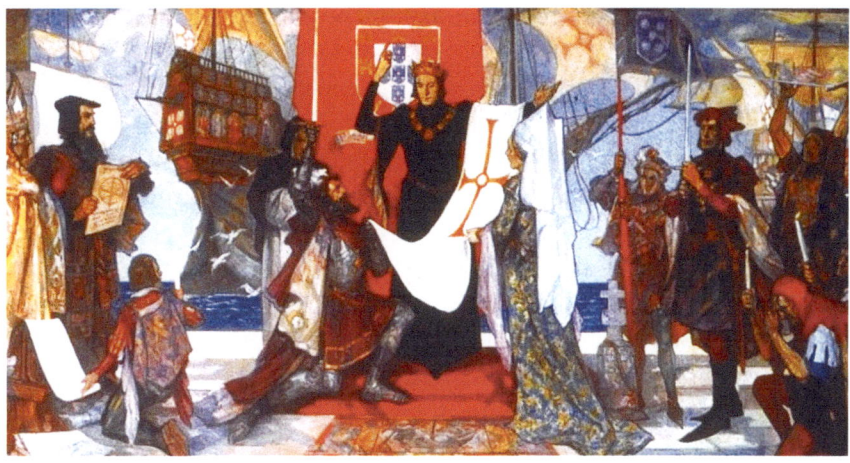

Figure 15.8 *Painting by John Henry Amshewitz (1882–1942)*

Portugal, featuring Zacuto presenting the explorer with his astronomical tables.

Stephen Hawking (1942–2018)

One, remember to look up at the stars and not down at your feet. Two, never give up work. Work gives you meaning and purpose, and life is empty without it. Three, if you are lucky enough to find love, remember it is there and don't throw it away.

Stephen Hawking[29]

Stephen Hawking an English theoretical physicist and **cosmologist**, held prestigious appointments in cosmology and mathematics at the University of Cambridge, Oxford University and California Institute of Technology. Hawking was the recipient of numerous academic and international awards. His mother is quoted as saying: "Stephen always had a strong sense of wonder, I could see that the stars would draw him".[30]

He was a popular author, and while his revolutionary work in physics and cosmology pushed the boundaries of science, he also made the knowledge

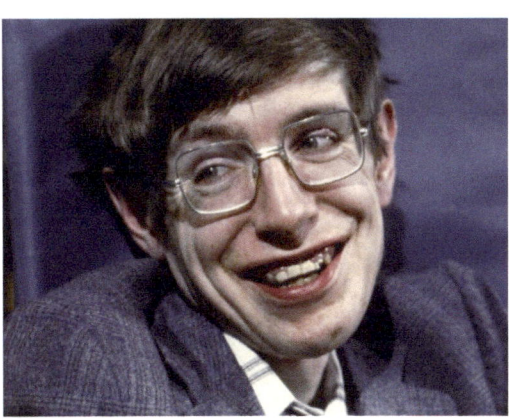

Figure 15.9 *Stephen Hawking (1942–2018*

accessible to the general public through more simplified books, such as, *A Brief History of Time*.[31]

Hawking's main achievement was to explain the beginning of the universe (cosmology) by combining the general theory of relativity with quantum mechanics. By this union, which replaces real time with imaginary time, the history of the universe becomes a **four-dimensional curved surface** with no boundary. In his research of black holes Hawking proposed that unlike the prevailing belief, all is not lost when an object enters a black hole. Its information is stored in 2D form within an outer boundary known as the "event horizon." Hawking claimed he could **think in 11 dimensions** and was convinced that time travel could be possible because of the hidden dimensions in the universe.

Hawkins challenged Newton's premises that God created the universe, claiming that because of singularity, there was nothing before the Big Bang and the universe was created spontaneously. He gave an analogy to the **Earth's South Pole**, where real time begins and holds to the laws of physics but south of the South Pole, there is nothing.

At age 21, Hawking was diagnosed with amyotrophic lateral sclerosis (ALS) and over the years he lost use of all of his muscles, was confined to a wheelchair and had to use a voice synthesiser. He later claimed the disease helped his scientific and publishing career.

*"Before my condition was diagnosed, I had been **very bored with life**,"* he said. *"There had not seemed to be anything worth doing."*[32]

Hawkins was finally able to **defy gravity**. In 2007, while visiting the Kennedy Space Centre in Florida, he was flown on a modified Boeing 727, during which he experienced weightlessness and was temporarily freed from his wheelchair.

Jacob

Biblical Jacob has two major themes in his life: **Time and work**.[33] He is the younger twin, born after his brother Esau, and therefore did not receive either blessing or the best inheritance. He spent most of his early life trying to **reverse time** and become the first born, which he eventually managed to do by deceiving his brother and father. Later in the story, he falls in love with the beautiful Rachel, but to gain her hand he must work hard for seven years. His love compresses time, and the seven years seem like a few days to him. Due to his intense love, Jacob is living in the continuous present moment, and the passage of time is not a factor. However, just as he deceived his father, Jacob is deceived, and rather than marrying his beloved Rachel, he is tricked into marrying her older sister, Leah, another

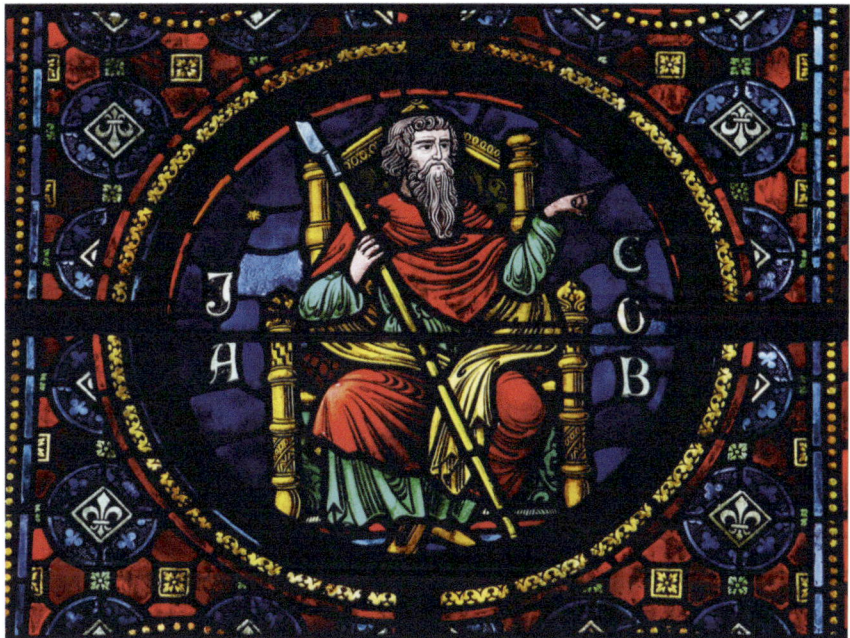

Figure 15.10 *Jacob*

time reversal trick. Again, he must work for seven years, which now appears infinitely longer. Finally, he marries Rachel, but he must work for seven more long tedious years to gain freedom. From his story we learn the lesson of time and work; **beloved work is timeless**, **while despised work drags on forever.**

Like Superman, Jacob is incredibly strong. He can lift a huge stone off a well, a task which usually requires several men. He is also able to wrestle with an **extra-terrestrial** angel and hold his own.

Galileo Galilei (1564–1642)

Mentioned in the proving, he was an Italian astronomer, mathematician, physicist, philosopher, and professor who made pioneering observations of nature with long-lasting implications for the study of physics. Galileo studied gravity, speed and velocity, the principle of relativity, inertia, and projectile motion, and he also worked in applied science and technology.[34]

Johannes Kepler (1571–1630)

Mentioned in the proving, he was a German astronomer, mathematician, astrologer, natural philosopher, and writer on music. Best known for his laws of planetary motion, he defended the Copernican heliocentric astronomy.[35]

Albert Einstein (1879–1933)

Mentioned in the proving and plenty of his quotes are included in the book already. He might belong to the fifth or further dimensions.[36]

The 14th Dali Lama (1935–)

He is mentioned in the proving and made an appearance in a blinded meditation proving the class did before the real proving. There are many references to Tibetan Buddhism in the proving. Other than that, I have no idea if he fits the Krypton bill.[37]

Waking dream of sitting alone on a vast plateau, and the Dalai Lama came to me grinning. He talked about a state of fresh virgin, unaltered by even a hair's breadth of concept.

References

1 Superman Biography and Superman Facts. *Superhero Stuff*. Available online at: https://www.superherostuff.com/biographies/supermanbio.html (accessed July 17, 2023).

2 Anon. Christopher Reeve: The Life of the Man of Steel. *Aruma*. Available online at: http://tinyurl.com/4t3urkj4 (accessed July 17, 2023).

3 Anon. Riddler. *The Batman Universal Wiki*. Available online at: http://tinyurl.com/mrcez2zw (accessed July 17, 2023).

4 DaVinci L. *Brainy Quote*. Available online at: http://tinyurl.com/yf6cakn5 (accessed July 18, 2023).

5 DaVinci L. *Brainy Quote*. Available online at: http://tinyurl.com/y2mydvr3 (accessed July 18, 2023).

6 Da Vinci – The Genius: The Renaissance Man. *Museum of Science*. Available online at: http://tinyurl.com/nhstc5fb (accessed July 17, 2023).

7 Mona Lisa's Hidden Symbols? *CBS News*, January 12, 2011. Available online at: http://tinyurl.com/yn9v5rb9 (accessed July 17, 2023).

8 Anon. Researchers Prove Leonardo da Vinci was Ambidextrous. *Physics*, April 9, 2019. Available online at: http://tinyurl.com/5n6nzr6s (accessed July 17, 2023).

9 Anon. The Vitruvian Man by Leonardo Da Vinci. Available online at: http://tinyurl.com/4dfd8v4p (accessed July 17, 2023).

10 Campbell County Health Group, Gillette WY. *Sleeping Like a Genius*, September 1, 2022. Available online at: http://tinyurl.com/rpvrby34 (accessed July 17, 2023).

11 Fluckiger S. Leonardo da Vinci and Animal Rights: 500 Years Ahead of His Time. *Petauk*, April 23, 2019. Available online at: http://tinyurl.com/38raynx7 (accessed July 17, 2023).

12 Copernicus N. *Brainy Quote*. Available online at: http://tinyurl.com/3s4uvuht (accessed July 18, 2023).

13 Copernicus N. *Brainy Quote*. Available online at: http://tinyurl.com/4puf56pp (accessed July 18, 2023).

14 Editors at History.com E. Nicolaus Copernicus. *History*. Available online at: http://tinyurl.com/dbket7c2 (accessed July 17, 2023).

15 Westman R. Nicolaus Copernicus. *Britannica*. Available online at: http://tinyurl.com/v7wybw98 (accessed July 17, 2023).

16 Carroll L. *Goodreads: Lewis Carroll Quotes*. Available online at: http://tinyurl.com/ypteceb2 (accessed July 18, 2023).

17 Carroll L. *Goodreads: Lewis Carroll Quotes*. Available online at: http://tinyurl.com/32snzzcm (accessed January 29, 2024).

18 Carroll L. *Goodreads: Lewis Carroll Quotes*. Available online at: http://tinyurl.com/4xay9ema (accessed January 29, 2024).

19 Green R. Lewis Carroll. *Britannica*, July 7, 2023. Available online at: http://tinyurl.com/3f3nkzyv (accessed July 17, 2023).

20 Beggs S. 11 Fascinating Facts About Lewis Carrol. *Mental Floss,* April 5, 2018. Available online at: http://tinyurl.com/yeuc7d4u (assessed July 17, 2023).

21 Carroll L. Solitude Poem. *Classical Literature*. Available online at: http://tinyurl.com/42cpv6jm (accessed January 30, 2024).

22 Gardner M. *Introduction to Alice's Adventures in Wonderland and Through the Looking-Glass*. Oxford: University Press, 2009.

23 Carroll L. The Walrus and the Carpenter. *Poetry Foundation*. Available online at: http://tinyurl.com/47nucts3 (accessed July 17, 2023).

24 Newton I. Gravity explains the motions of the planets, but it cannot explain who sets the planets in motion. Quote available online at: https://www.azquotes.com/quote/411519 (accessed July 18, 2023).

25 Buttar S. How Newton Changed the Course of History in One Year. *Secrets of the Universe*. Available online at: http://tinyurl.com/6vtnk2ju (accessed July 17, 2023).

26 Newton H. The Character of Sir Isaac Newton. *English Language and History*. Available online at: http://tinyurl.com/4yy4mz54 (accessed July 17, 2023).

27 Mindel N. Rabbi Abraham Zacuto. *Chabad*. Available online at: http://tinyurl.com/2nfaca8p (accessed July 17, 2023).

28 The Lusiads. *Britannica*. Available online at: http://tinyurl.com/yww4mbke (accessed July 17, 2023).

29 Hawking SW. *Stephen Hawkins Quotes*. Available online at: http://tinyurl.com/4vhmw4p6 (accessed January 29, 2024).

30 Anon. Stephen Hawking. *Biography*. Available online at: http://tinyurl.com/4s97j5fb (accessed July 17, 2023).

31 Hawking SW. *A Brief History of Time*. New York NY: Bantam Dell Publishing Group, 1988.

32 Hawking SW. *My Brief History*. New York NY: Bantam Books, 2013.

33 Jacob. *New World Encyclopedia*. Available online at: http://tinyurl.com/2naed2j9 (accessed July 17, 2023).

34 Galileo Galilei. *Britannica*. Available online at: http://tinyurl.com/5n7bphkb (accessed July 17, 2023).

35 Johannes Kepler. *Britannica*. Available online at: http://tinyurl.com/ykts7zy4 (accessed July 17, 2023).

36 Albert Einstein. *Britannica*. Available online at: http://tinyurl.com/p553e6xd (accessed July 17, 2023).

37 Dalai Lama. *Britannica*. Available online at: http://tinyurl.com/2fnhr7ex (accessed July 17, 2023).

16

KRYPTOGRAPHY

Nobody quite knows what is going on. Things are not what they seem.

> Kepler counting, Rabbi blessing
> Moon and sun revolve
> Six and thirty puzzles here
> That you cannot re-solve

Krypton is a remedy that speaks in codes, riddles and ciphers. One cannot simply leave a code without trying to crack it. Riddles often have more than one answer, so here are just a few attempts from myself, and a few for you to sharpen your mind on. Even if you are not interested in unravelling these enigmas, it will give you some insight into how the Kryptic mind works. Let's begin with the riddle which opened this book:

There was a joke when I woke Four cons = it was cryptic. Con cave was the cave a con? A "C" is a quarter of an "8". Dismember the * and you get four C's.

My crack: The number four is integral to this proving, fourth period and chakra. Cryptic = Krypton. But a crypt can also be a cave, which is concave, as well as meaning a code, or a con (a fraud). If a C is concave or convex depending which way the C is facing, they are mirror images of each other. C is also Carbon, which has a strong relationship to Krypton – it is in the middle column the 4th element in the second period, and thus opposite the nobles. Place 4 C's together (One on top of each other and mirror image) and you get an 8. You can dismember 8 back into 4 C's. The proving has several references to dismembering. The * sign is an asterisk, the star (from Greek *asteriskos*, 'little star'), which you can draw with 4 C's placed back-to-back. The keyboard asterisk is located on the 8 key.

Numbers

The numbers 3, 4, 8, 9, 12, 36, 72, 90, 108 and 360 are significant in Krypton and relate to atomic numbers of elements, degrees or segments of a circle, longitude meridians, hours, the four heart quadrants and the heart rate at rest.

Only seeing male patients today – ages 4, 8, 12 and 36. A series.

$3 \times 4 = 12 \times 3 = 36 =$ Krypton.

I was told about Venus's 3% tilt – if the Earth equaled one, then Venus equalled 0.72. Also, Venus is 108 million km from the sun.

Other than the astrological significance of this statement, let's play with the numbers. 72 is twice 36, 36 × 3 makes 108.

90 + 18 = 108. After the seven days, what then?

18, the atomic number of Argon, also signifies the Tree of Life in Hebrew. 90 in Hebrew signifies the righteous one, Tsadik, also meaning upright person, he who stands at 90 to the earth. At all times there are 36 of these people on earth.

The combination of the 18 + 90, the Tree of Life and the upright person gives 108. This is a sacred number for many traditions, as well as mathematically significant.[1] Of course, 108 is the same as 18, only with a significant nothing added in between.

The overlap between Einstein and Kepler is to do with Carbon 12 and generations of stars. There are 12 constellations positrons and neutrinos combining – fastness.
C12 – C120 – which generation?
Different chains – proton-proton- or carbon
This is to liberate us from repetition
0 with 1 in the middle = ten

In 1961 the isotope carbon-12 was selected to replace oxygen as the standard relative to which all atomic weights are measured.

The proton–proton chain, or p–p chain, is one of two known sets of nuclear fusion reactions by which stars convert hydrogen to helium. The CNO cycle, the other known reaction, is suggested by theoretical models to dominate in stars with masses greater than about 1.3 times that of the Sun.

0 with 1 in the middle = 10. 1 or 0, line or circle, represent linear or circular thinking.

Dream about 12 gifts, and the 13th gift was sleep. Perhaps we sleep until we're sexually awakened. There was a conversation about 12 years between Keppler and Newton, and they were discussing the word "scale" and coming up with four meanings – scale was a balance, climb, proportion and covering.

The 12 pearls refer to the 12 gates of Jerusalem

Scale also means measurement, which is an important aspect of Krypton, the main gift of the Tree of Knowledge.

I was dreaming about the 7 stars of the Great Bear and their notes and colours. There were 7 rays, candlesticks, angels, spirits of God, seals, hills, thunders, veils of initiation and pomegranate petals. Jacob – truth or peace? Ten sayings. It was about the King of Edom. Segol + chesed. 613 parts? 12 shevet. The Hebrew 4th letter "D" has an angle of 90 degrees. It is two doors to the world. The top one opening to the North minus reason. This is given to us, no mind all heart, freely given.

My Crack: Seven noble gases, chakras, and days of creation.
613 body parts and commandments in Jewish tradition.[2]
No mind, all heart, one side of Krypton, with all heart and no mind. The other side is all brain no heat.
For Jacob, see Chapter 15 Theoretical Krypton cases. The first King of Edom was Esau, his brother. Edom later prevented the 12 tribes (shevet = tribe) from passing through their land.
D is the fourth Hebrew letter. It means door of gateway, and has an angle of 90%. There are two gateways at the poles.

Four

The number 4 is a powerful symbol in the world of Krypton. It not only relates to its fourth period, but also provides some insight into other key aspects such as quarters and chakras.

Thoughts about the heart. Hearts are quartered like the 4 quarters of Jerusalem. A new Jerusalem was built using the same stone. Blake was talking about the fourfold division of Jerusalem – every part and thing and person is in 4 quarters.
Wrote 'cauterised' as 'quarterised'.
A circle within a square could be more dynamic than a square within a circle.

Measured time is chopped up and quarterised into four, creating right angles which are rigid beliefs. Rather than our inner self being round time and fluid, we get internal square time and concept.

Dreams of crypts and things being cryptic and coptic, of Egypt and Osiris. Four faces but five lines.

36

Dream about feet and shoes. If I was European, they would be size 36 but in Great Britain they are size 4.

Woke after a dream. Fish were multiplying – now there were 139, or were there 136? with one swimming/spinning so fast that it looked like 4.

Dreamt four of us were out to eat. When we came to pay with notes, the bill was £36. We gave £50 and we got a £53 or £54 note back.

JS: note the atomic number of Xenon is 54.

Magic Square of the Sun (Sol)[3]

In my mind's eye I was seeing magic squares and how our sun is 6 × 6 which is 36 and Venus is 7 × 7.

6	32	3	34	35	1
7	11	27	28	8	30
19	14	16	15	23	24
18	20	22	21	17	13
25	29	10	9	26	12
36	5	33	4	2	31

Figure 16.1 *Magic Square of the Sun*

The numbers associated with the Sun are 6, 36, 111, and 666. This is because:

Each row and column of the magic square contains six numbers.

The square contains 36 numbers total, ranging from 1 to 36.

Each row, column and diagonal add up to 111.

All of the numbers in the square add up to 666.

The divine names associated with The Sun all have numerological values of 6 or 36. These values are calculated by writing out the names in Hebrew and then adding up the value of each included letter, as each Hebrew letter can represent both a sound and a numerical value.

Word puzzles

Voices Karnak it's not the ark but the arc – arc lights, alignments Carnac.

Here we see the play between the linear K and the circular C. Both Karnak in Egypt and Carnac in France have monuments with star alignments. Arc means to curve, and arc lights were the earliest form of electric light, now made with krypton and xenon instead of Carbon.

In Eddington's experiment in which he proved Einstein's theories with measurements from **seven stars** in good visibility, he gave the deflection as 1.98(+/–) 0.16 **arc** seconds.

Words letters codes

ne on

arg on

krypt on

The lights are on – He

I needed to know what "on" meant in Greek.

Neutral Greek words tend to end in -on. The neutral ending 'on' in Krypton refers to a thing/something, so Krypton would be a hidden thing, something hidden. 'On' also means lights ON, which happens when nobles are pumped with electricity.

All I could hear was 'To be or not to be', that is the question, whether it is nobler … mind. The words were Beheaded, Betrayed, Believed, Becalmed, Beware, Because. I was then given four definitions of what Be means: To have existence. To exist in the world of fact whether physical or mental. To become. To remain.

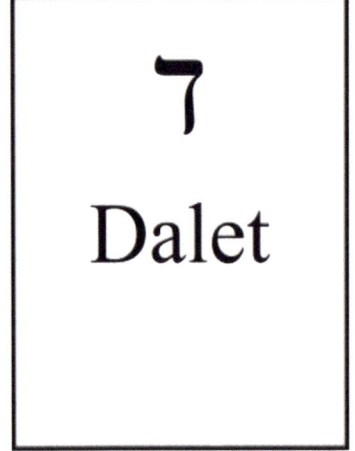
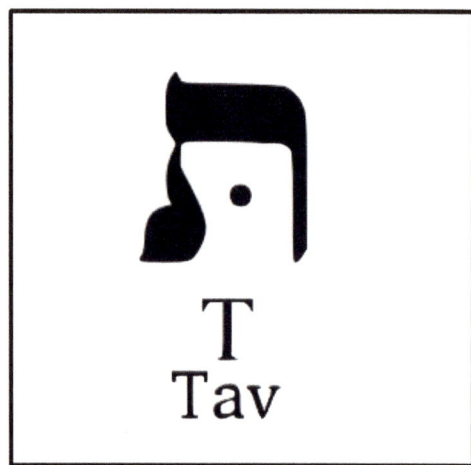

Figure 16.2 *The Hebrew letter Dalet*   ***Figure 16.3*** *The Hebrew letter Tavv*

To be or to re, this is the question: Be in the dynamic, spiritual, continuous present moment, or become becalmed and stuck in repetitive gravitational karma, and be beheaded and betrayed. Beware.

Hebrew looks like a foreign language.
D + D = T

The letter D is equivalent to the letter Dalet in Hebrew. It is the fourth letter and signifies a door (delet means door). It is composed of two lines at 90° to each other.

If we join two Dalet letters together (one reversed) we get the letter 'Tav', meaning T. It is the last letter of the Hebrew alphabet, signifying completion, and the number 400. Hence D + D = T.

Sensation heartbeat like a drum. Then the 'r' went out of 'heart' to make 'heat', the 'h' went to make 'eat', then it could either be 'et' or 'at' – the 'et' being Hebrew.

Et and At, same as be and re.

Mirrors, opposites

Krypton represents the mirror between the top and bottom halves of the periodic table. Below Krypton we live in an upside-down world. Here all things reverse, preventing us from finding the true way home unless we can see through the deception. Meanwhile our brain must invert all that our eyes see.

Passed through Oldhill, for which the sign read Hold Ill (holding on to being ill – the security of having symptoms) and at Snow Hill, the sign read Now Hills.

Old hill and Now hill may relate to 'on top of the mountain' and 'in the eternal present', connected to eternal time, the lofty state of Krypton. Hold ill means holding on to our disease, that which we do in chronic disease on the slippery slope to oblivion.

On own now, now own one, no own now, own one/won, we won?

In this word play we see the opposition of the eternal present 'now' and the temporary selfishness of 'own'. Can we win if we own?

Dream of reversal of the seven days.

If, from our chronic disease perspective we are looking through the mirror, the sequence of the days should be reversed, starting from the Sabbath day of rest on the first day, on to the creation of man in the second and progressing towards the creation of light in the seventh. Does it make sense? Not to the way our mind works, but then we live behind the mirror. In the world beyond, water flows upwards, and the correct sequence of writing is right to left.
(See Bromium and Kali in Chapter 17.)

The river Jordan flowed the other way.
Writing right to left.
I was witnessing the birth of letters seeing them coming into being in English and Hebrew. Hebrew starts at the back of the book.
In the Tarot the Wheel of Fortune is No 21 the opposite to the Hanged Man No 12.

Let's examine the opposition of these two Tarot cards. Both relate to time and change, but while the Wheel of Fortune card indicates timely and positive change, the Hanged Man is difficult, slow, and unclear, and may mean giving up part of yourself. In the first you are on top of the time cycle, in the second time is controlling you.

Codes for you to crack

Here are a few more proving puzzles which I am leaving to you to dwell on.

Quasars – blue and compact emit a very strong radio wave, stronger than is possible. It's to do with us not understanding why there is 30 something % more matter in the universe than we can calculate.

2H atoms collide to make heavy hydrogen a 3rd makes HE3 Beryllium when they separate again. Another He makes He4 + 2H released stable Helium very fast timeless.

Waking dream: of being really happy and asked whether it was happy with an 'i' or a 'y'. I was told I was happy with an 'i' i.e. 'hapi'. He helped resurrect Osiris by suckling him. Hapy with a 'y' was one of Horus's, who was one of Osiris' sons. This son was in charge of the jar with the lungs in it. I was told it was an honour for Man to fall into the Nile and be eaten by a crocodile. I was told crocodiles are good because they eat rough (both not smooth and not good quality) fish, and that the sun energy was too warm and dry me out.

Dream I was a child given a book of tides. The face of a clock was looking like Hebrew letters. The word 'ALEF' came up, and the letters changed around. I wondered, in English 'a etc' why not have two vowels together? Like 'leave' – which means either to go or to produce leaves. I was told it was because one made two. Were the letters open at the back or the front? The word 'fairy'.

Dream I couldn't find the calendar for this year or month. I was trying to explain to him an ancient calendar. All the figures were ancient knowledge, but they had this year's date above them. He was only seeing half. The figures were 3.35 so it must have been 6.70 or 67. He was not complete as he had not tail.

Dream. I said 11 more things, like dawn, yawn, fawn, bawn, hawn, lawn, mawn, wawn, pawn, sawn and tawn, but I was aware that we spell most of them with "orn".

Seeing the ALEF as a big soup of shades and universal sounds.

10 in Hebrew means fire from above. We no longer move in single figures. cipher.

References

1 Mulla L. Significance of the Number 108, *Numerology*. Available online at: http://tinyurl.com/ens7xx8e (accessed July 17, 2023).
2 The 613 Commandments. *Jewish Virtual Library*. Available online at: http://tinyurl.com/3b723h9m (accessed July 17, 2023).
3 Planetary Magical Squares. *Learn Religions*. Available online at: http://tinyurl.com/zy6a27zj (accessed July 17, 2023).

17

RELATED REMEDIES

I will not be discussing the whole fourth row of remedies, as there are too many. You might want to read about some of these remedies in my article *Tinker, Tailer, Soldier, Spy: A Voyage on the Fourth Highway to Krypton*.[1] Instead, I will do the first and last, Kali and Bromium. Or perhaps, now that we are looking through the mirror, Bromium and Kali!

Potassium, Kali metallicum, Element 19

I will begin with Potassium, gateway to the fourth row, from a remarkable mini-mediation proving from Camilla. Kali metallicum has not been potentised, because, like all group one elements, it reacts immediately with water and sugar. However, as this was a meditation proving, we were able to do it. The proving was single blind, Camilla did not know the substance.

Image of a dark alleyway with a car coming with head lights on. Like from a crime movie or series.

A dark violent place. People with hoods come out. They take a body out in a body bag.

Very strong powerful energy hard to resist. It feels you have to go to sleep to avoid it.

I feel like I'm swinging like a vertigo. Swinging almost falling asleep. Like flipping into another world.

Like the dream world, the underworld. Feels like if you just let go and lose control you will just be in it. But there is something menacing about it, like a mafia. I feel as if I could just flip into a dream, very close the dream world. I do for one split second.

Obs. Her eyes are closed, nodding off, heavy. Speaking heavily.

'I dreamt something but forgot. Dream while speaking'.

I have to open my eyes not to slip into that world.

This is like the stage in between life and death. No death and no life. Or no life and no death?

Like going lucid. I feel weird in my head.

I keep having tiny little dreams. Now a reunion with family members. Then I met a girlfriend of my stepdaughter who is here in this weird world. They fell out and now they are ready to give it a go again and make up.

I'm talking about dreams, but I can't explain it. I don't know what I'm talking about.

Nodding off again. Dreaming.

I've never had this kind of flipping in and out ... like totally on the border between the two, dream and reality. Between the underworld or dream world and the awake world.

I feel totally knocked out. I can't keep to either reality, flipping from one to the other and back. I can't keep here and can't keep there. Waking in the dream world and back coming again.

I can't grasp the dreams, can't hold them.

Dreams of family members, saying goodbye or meeting again. Not staying together. A point of disconnection. The point of disconnection or re-connection after disconnection.

Feel like I'm drugged. Eyes rolling in my sockets. Out of it. This is like fragmentation.

Feel like I'm someone else I had a dream of being someone else and I just wanted to let go and die.

As if you are on the brink and if you let go it pulls you into a void.

This is very heavy, very, very heavy!! Talking in slow motion and deep slurred voice.

It's like a magnetic pull, not magnetic, like a pull but not gravity.

A pull to the underworld, to the abyss. Like touch and go.

So heavy and so tired.

It's not a pull into heavenly light, it's a pull to the underground. Heavy. Body and bones feel heavy, head heavy. Nodding off. This is not nice, not a nice place to be.

Again, I had this Mrs. Robinson song: 'Any way you look at it you lose' But this time in a deep slow heavy voice. Now I can hear 'Slip sliding away' in my head.

I would not want to go to that abyss. Too dark and scary, a pull, it wants to suck you in.

'Slip sliding away ... and headed home again'.

Dream stepdaughter holding baby daughter, carrying her, holding her.

Fragmentation. Strong fall into the abyss. The black hole. I don't want to go there. I don't think you can find your way back if you go there. Having meaningless fragments of dreams. I am just at the cusp of sleep and awake, on the brink of going in or staying out. Seeing black shadows in the corner of my eyes, a bit afraid. Making me nervous to be at the gate. Heavy,

heavy, heavy. I need ice cream to get me out of this. I don't want to go into this, it's just black, a black vortex. I am scared because if I go in, I might not get out. It's a journey downwards through the dream. But this abyss is the real thing. It is not a facade or a delusion. The vortex is the real thing. The pull is through the dream world. You have to go through the dream world to get there. Like maybe when you die you have fragments of very fast dreams before the vortex suck you in. The vortex is real. Reality, dream then vortex. This remedy is at the bottom of the world, then vortex. The vortex is deep with seemingly no end, but there is light at the end of the tunnel, and it flips back up. Really, it's not that far down.

Dreaming, something about circumcision.

The following is a list of some related rubrics from Kali carbonicum.[2] * represents degree. Carbs are usually the most neutral salt. Note that these are not exactly the conventional homoeopathic Kali carb essence, which, in my opinion, is limiting.

mind; ANGUISH (371) ***
mind; ANXIETY; future, about; disease, and of her *
mind; CLINGING; mother, to *
mind; DELUSIONS, imaginations; devil, devils *
mind; DELUSIONS, imaginations; die; about to *
mind; DELUSIONS, imaginations; disease; has; incurable, has *
mind; DELUSIONS, imaginations; emptiness, of; behind him on turning around *
mind; DELUSIONS, imaginations; figures, sees; old repulsive persons, which fill her with fear, in hysteria ***
mind; DELUSIONS, imaginations; images, phantoms, sees; frightful *
mind; DELUSIONS, imaginations; people, some one; ugly *
mind; DELUSIONS, imaginations; spectres, ghosts, spirits, sees *
mind; DELUSIONS, imaginations; vermin; crawl about, sees *
mind; DESPAIR; recovery, of *
mind; DREAMS; danger; forms, of, passing by **
mind; DREAMS; dead; people, of ***
mind; DREAMS; death, of; approaching *
mind; DREAMS; death, of; relatives *
mind; FEAR; visions of old repulsive persons, from, in hysteria ***
mind; DREAMS; falling; high places, of, from height *
mind; DREAMS; family, own *
mind; FEAR; agoraphobia *
mind; FEAR; alone, being ****
mind; FEAR; alone, being; die, lest he ***

mind; FEAR; death, of ****
mind; FEAR; failure, of; business or work, in ***
mind; FEAR; forsaken, of being ***
mind; FEAR; narrow place, in, claustrophobia *

Jeremy's comments

After the magic moment of Argon's eternal childhood, Kali begins the descent into the underworld, which will culminate with Krypton crossing into the other side. In and out our consciousness dips, slip sliding away from life into the dream world. Or is it out of the dream world and into life?

So interesting that the song Mrs. Robinson was a theme of Camilla's Argon proving, symbolising childhood vs maturity. Now it continues, but in a heavier way. Once you cross over to the chronic dark side, you lose any which way you go. "Slip Sliding Away" was the song Camilla and I got in the Krypton proving. Obviously, Paul Simon was here.

The theme of the family connecting and disconnecting is interesting, as the family connection and disconnection is well known in the Kali's, especially prominent in Kali carbonicum and Kali phosphoricum. Obviously, this is the brink between upper and lower world, wake and dreaming, family and vortex. Finally, circumcision is an act of locking the male out of the heavenly dream world and into our physical world (women do this automatically).

Bromium: Element 35

Here is the next mini-proving, this time of Bromium. This is the element 35, the last element before Krypton.

I yawned and felt my mouth was a huge cavity, huge!

As if my jaw opened really wide, not possible that someone has such an open mouth and a massive cavity.

Oh God, my mouth is so huge. Like I'm all mouth. I have to yawn all the time, and when I yawn my mouth is so big.

Now my eyes feel so big, weird.

Yawning wide. My mouth is huge and eyes huge, this is really good for people with lockjaw.

As if my eyes are huge and staring. (Her eyes are open wide.)

I feel like I am all head, and my body is very small.

I feel like a whale with a huge mouth, but at the same time I feel like a microscopic creature with only two orifices, a huge mouth and eyes and nothing else. With a whale the mouth is proportionally Huge. How many teeth does a whale have? hundreds?

I feel like someone with really big eyes but innocent and childish.

Like a child with no idea what just hit you, someone screamed at you. Like when you are little, and you have big wide eyes because you take in everything around you, but you don't understand it all or put in context, some adults yell at you, you are so innocent and pure, you have no way to defend yourself, you don't know what hit you, disbelief, not understating, all eyes and mouth but no brain to understand , psychologise or theorise. You are wide-eyed innocent, and you have just been whacked and screamed at, and you have no idea what happened and what you are supposed to do, no tools to process it and no way to understand it. You can't even put an arm up to defend, or hide, or take cover, or leave the room, no experience, you were just slapped and screamed at for the first time, a shock, all wide eyed and can't comprehend what just happened, like the first abuse for a child. That is what it feels like.

Can happen to anyone, it may be adults that it has not happened to yet, where it takes days for the shock to sink in. Like falling from the heaven, the first smack of brutality.

Like a one- or two-celled creature, because the human complexity needs sophistication and language and experience, but when you are a little child or an Amazonian Indian you can't even comprehend any of that shit, because there is a purity and innocence.

Crying …

This is when innocence ends! And it is heartbreaking. And it happened to all of us, no one can escape it … maybe on a remote island where no abuser ever went.

Before the cerebral, you are all eyes and all mouth, and the brain has not developed yet, has not lived yet, no siblings, kindergarten, school or parent have messed you up yet.

It is all still oral. Food, sucking on the breast, eyes looking at the world in wonder. The oral phase?

And then it ends. A big grief. Suddenly you understand that it is not all good and not all safe.

It's a rude awakening. Even the people who love you the most will hurt you.

Could be what happens when your mother dies at a young age. Up to that point infinite trust …

Everything so lovely, so loved, so safe, then suddenly in one second all of that vanishes, you have to fend for yourself. Like when the angles fall. So sad.

We came onto this planet because we knew we would experience all of this, but you forget, so the shock is so brutal, every time so brutal because every time you forget.

But it has to happen because otherwise how will you live here. Not enough pure pacific islands.

It's like you have to swallow it, to go through all the reflexes, this is inevitable. No parent can protect their child from it, though they want to. Like when you see another child being horrible to yours, you recognize the shock on their face when some kid punches them, and you feel the pain because you recognise it, it's the inevitable ripping out of trusting innocence.

And every parent would rip their heart out to save their child from that, but you can't.

The pain of being alive. You can't protect them. Even if you don't whack them yourself someone else will.

It's the most devastating if it comes from those that love you the most, if someone else does it at least you can run to your parents. The ultimate betrayal is when it comes from your parents. Better off to be safe with a good home, safe haven. Then you can thrive, something they can count on. If they don't have that they have nothing, the world is just hostile.

Song playing in my head: 'The first cut is the deepest, baby I know'.

No one will tell you this in clinic, they won't remember it, happens before you have words and understanding and can give explanations, no one can put their finger on it. You are still a baby and you mum feeds you in the night, and one night she is so tired and exhausted, she groans and pushes you away, and that's it … its inevitable, no one can escape it. First grief, first pain. An adult can handle it because they know, but when you're little your eyes are wide open and innocent. Everything goes in, you don't know what whacked you. Every child needs someone safe that loves him completely and unconditionally. Unconditional love is the key to everything. Otherwise, people love you because you are smart or clever or pretty. But that is not why you should love anyone, you love someone because you love them, that is the only way love is. When you have that from someone, I love you because I love you, that is real love. Children feel that way from their parents. Loved full stop. That is the biggest gift you can give to your children or anyone. Love no matter what.

Some related rubrics from the Complete Repertory.[2]
* represents degree

mind; ANXIETY; dark, in *

  mind; ANXIETY; heart region ***

  mind; CARRIED; desires to be ***

  mind; CHILDREN; complaints in *

  mind; DELUSIONS, imaginations; images, phantoms, sees **

  mind; DELUSIONS, imaginations; jump, jumped; objects jump around floor *

  mind; DELUSIONS, imaginations; people, some one ***

  mind; DELUSIONS, imaginations; people, some one; behind him, someone, something is ***

  mind; DELUSIONS, imaginations; persecuted, that he is ***

  mind; DELUSIONS, imaginations; person; another in the room *

  mind; DELUSIONS, imaginations; stranger, strangers; sees ***

  mind; DREAMS; fights *

  mind; DREAMS; frightful, nightmare ***

  mind; DREAMS; murder ***

  mind; DREAMS; quarrels, strife ***

  mind; FEAR; behind him, that someone is *

  mind; FEAR; dark, of *

  mind; WEEPING, tearful mood; children, in *

  mind; WEEPING, tearful mood; looked at, when *

Jeremy's comments

An outstanding proving that dives deep into the secrets of Bromium, an innocent child a moment before the Krypton intellect takes over to analyse, deny, and protect the primal pain. However, this begs the question, is the innocent child with no intellect at the beginning of this period or at its end. Are we viewing the fourth period through the looking glass? That would place Kali standing on the precipice of a fall into darkness, at the gateway to the fifth period. Obviously from the number of protons and electrons the period proceeds from Kali to Brom, but the inner essence of the provings does not have to follow that theme. Food for thought.

Can the periodic table flow the other way after Krypton? Here is the proving:

Dream of reversal of the seven days.

The river Jordan flowed the other way.

Writing right to left.

I was witnessing the birth of letters seeing them coming into being in English and Hebrew. Hebrew starts at the back of the book.

Neon

There is a direct relationship between the nobles, and they may often follow each other well clinically.

Krypton seems to echo Neon, the second noble gas, in its connection to other planets, distant stars and galaxies. The second and fourth day of creation both deal with the skies.

Before falling asleep I moved to align myself directly with the stars through the sky window in my room. I joined the stars as I fell asleep. Krypton

I just long for some clear nights, so I can see my stars. If I could reconnect, then everything would be all right. Neon

Both remedies are related to numbers, especially even ones, 2, 4, 12, 36, etc.

One becomes two and two becomes one in order to create the universe. Krypton

I've always really liked odd numbers. I suddenly felt the capacity to be even. Even numbers were much more attractive. Neon

Cryptococcus

What's in a name? Another remedy of codes and riddles, all hidden in the crypt. I would say that cryptococcus is Krypton on acid. Or rather magic mushrooms.

Nobody quite knows what is going on. Things are not what they seem. Krypton

Things are not what they seem. Cryptococcus

References

1   Jeremy and friends. Available online at: https://www.patreon.com/JEREMYSHERR
2   van Zandvoort, R. *Complete Repertory*, 2019.

18

KRYPTON MMM: NIGHT TIME

Introduction

> By curving flat spacetime,
> God created the universe.
> Planets, red dwarfs, black holes, suns,
> Moons
> So if you wish to create
> don't shy away from
> Bending
> linear logic into curved magic.
> Tis an ill wind that blows no mind.

This is a theoretical and philosophical article. Nevertheless, it is all true, in a particular corner of the universe. The question is, is that the corner we are in now?

As befitting an MMM potency chapter, I will synthesise scientific ideas, proving data, poetry, mythologies, and metaphor into a meta concept concerning different forms of time, the periodic table, health and disease, sleep, dreams and homoeopathy. My advantage is that I have very pertinent information from my noble gas provings, information that has never been available previously. Provings are a window to a deeper understanding of the universe.

The ideas I am using from physics are all documented by accomplished scientists, yet they are often unconventional. Who cares. Homoeopathy is unconventional, but nevertheless true.

A Grief History of Time

> *Time is an illusion.*
>
> Albert Einstein[1]

As Krypton deals with the concept of time to a large extent, in the following chapter I will discuss the nature of time, and particularly its implications for sleep. I hope it will become clear why I am calling this a *Grief History of Time.* So no, it is not a typo.

I will compare the evolution of time to stages of the periodic table and specifically to the noble gases. If you have followed this series, you will have perceived that the noble gases act as mirrors, each reversing concepts from the previous period into the next period and a new reality. Here are some examples.

Helium

I felt the connection via a mirror.

If two humans look into a mirror, do they see the same, or opposite, or reverse sides?

Complete the web. Enter the mirror, dive into watery reflection.

Neon

Dream of me finding a broad-rimmed hand mirror.

Krypton

H and A are the same in mirror image.

Xenon

There were odd sloping floors, and mirrors which appeared to cause people who were walking to change appearance and direction. A teenage boy seemed to be partially through a mirror and then stretched out from the mirror, as though the mirror was controlling and rejecting him.

It is said the true prophets prophesise by looking through the mirror[2] and that the gateway to higher truth is through paradox. I said that! Nevertheless, English author Richard Le Gallienne wrote,[3]

A paradox is a truth standing on its head in order to attract attention.

But I personally think paradox only applies to jumping to a higher level of truth. Reversing concepts allows us a glimpse into the consciousness of the realities above and below us.

This applies also to the concept of time. Thus, there is a Helium time, which will reverse into Neon time, and then crossover and mirror itself into Argon, Krypton, Xenon, Radon and Luciferium time. Each of these time frames presents a different reality.

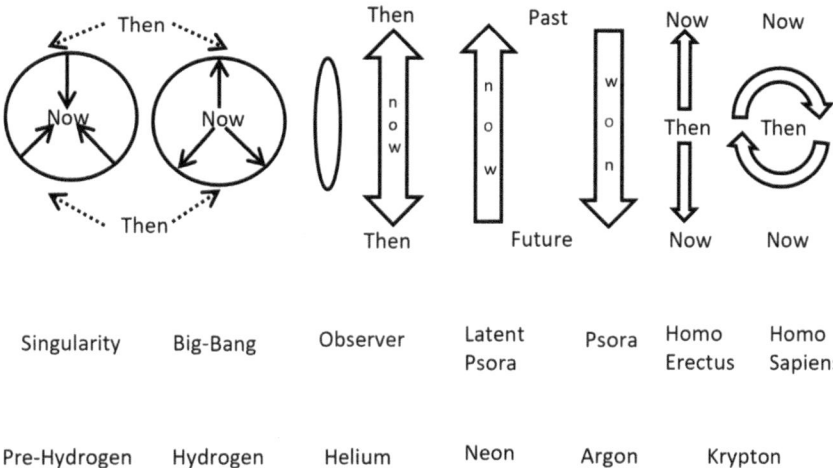

	n o w	n o w	w o n		

Singularity Big-Bang Observer Latent Psora Psora Homo Erectus Homo Sapiens

Pre-Hydrogen Hydrogen Helium Neon Argon Krypton

Figure 18.1 *Now then. A Grief History of Time*

Figure 18.1 depicts the history of time and its distortion through the lenses and mirrors of human observation and perception. I will explain it one step at a time.

We will start the journey in Argon time, because we believe we live in the third dimension, and imagine this to be all of reality. From this perspective we visualize an 'arrow of time', a corridor of rolling events stretching from a past lying behind us to a future extending ahead of us, on which we relentlessly march from childhood to death (Figure 18.2). This narrow temporal passage could be called a 'time prison'. It can also be called **Psora**. We consider this to be the only time frame, but that is a delusion, as it is not the only form of time.

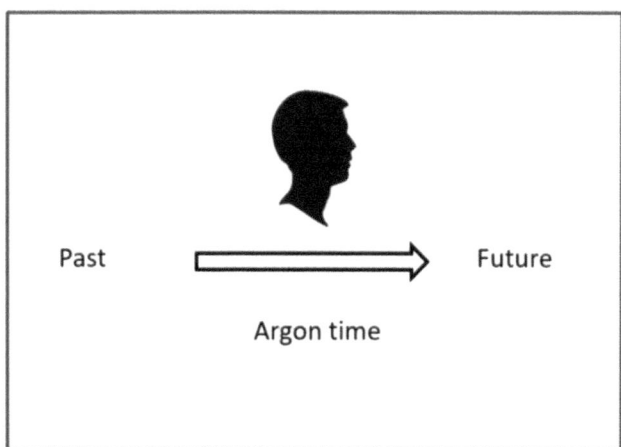

Figure 18.2 *Argon time. Looking forward to it*

Let's take a step upwards into the Neon period. Neon represents primary or latent Psora, and it is also confined to an 'arrow of time'. Neon perceives this time corridor:

Feel out of control, as if time is moving relentlessly and remorselessly forward, and I'm stuck behind, unable to keep up. Panic, guilt, constant anxiety that I won't get it all done.

Prior to taking the remedy, I felt too far in the future without realizing it. I feel as if I have **taken a step back** and am in the **here and now**. (curative)

It's as if I've lost the thread with the past that connects all past days together. It has dissolved. I seem to be more in the moment and less hurried. (curative)

It is the dissolving of time into the here and now that proves these symptoms to be curative.

However, as we step through the looking glass, the direction of Neon's time arrow reverses, and is now from a past in front of us to a future behind (Figure 18.3).

I remembered the incidences in dreams in the reverse order in which they happened.

At this stage, the 'arrow of time' is moving from future to past, just as for the Aymaras, members of a little-known culture of the Americas centred in the ancient city of Tiahuanac, who experience time in reverse.[4] In contrast to most modern Psoric civilizations, to the Aymara the past appears before them, and the future lies behind. They claim that they can see the past;

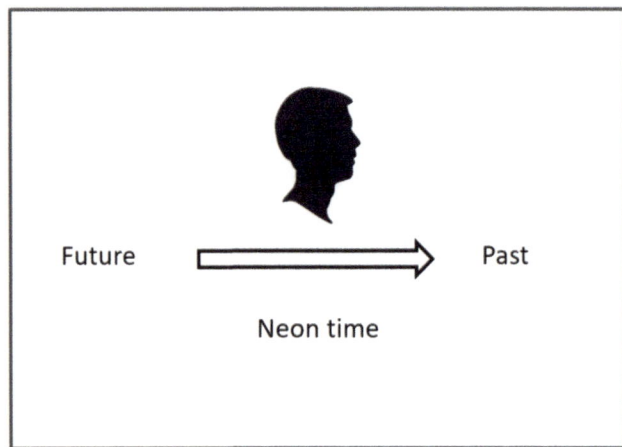

Figure 18.3 *Neon time. Back to the future*

therefore, it must be situated in front of their eyes, whereas the unknown future lurks in the shadows behind. Makes sense. They face the past with their backs to the future, so time flows backwards through them. Like other aboriginal tribes, they live in 'dream time' which to us seems naïve and childish. This is latent Psora; a confined delusion of reality, like that of a Neon newborn child stuck in an 'arrow of time'. But not as deluded as our Psoric, three-dimensional Argon 'reality'. The Aymara don't believe what they can't see. We do (e.g., man landed on the moon).

Now we travel up to the first period. How was time before Psora, in the spiritual period of Helium, the soul, before we are confined to our bodies and the delusion of an 'arrow of time'? Helium time is not linear, a simple forwards and backwards motion restricted to a one-direction passageway. Rather, Helium space-time time is helical, and turns in a spiral movement with now in the centre and the *then* in the periphery (Figure 18.4). Several physicists and philosophers agree that space-time may flow in a helical shape, or even in a double helix.[5,6]

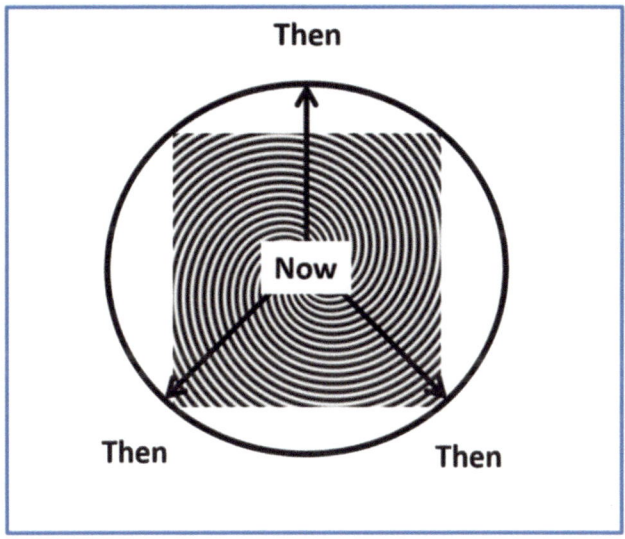

Figure 18.4 Helium circular time. Now now

From Helium

A spiral maze. The spiral of the self and the search for self, symbolising the wandering of the soul circling inward and outward ... Your spiralling dance through life.

I had an inner vision of my thumbprint, and then I saw labyrinths and maze patterns.

Then I have an image of spiralling downwards ... I pass through many flashes of other lives and experiences that I am simultaneously living, and passing through to get to this point of birth, this point of incarnation. And here I will stop for a 'time' (and how illusory is time?!) before I pass onwards in my soul's journey.

In the first period, time consciousness is *now-centric*: the present is in the middle, and from here time travels in all directions. There is only one central *here-now*, but there are infinite peripheral *there-thens*. As now is in the centre, forward time travels towards the future past (or to coin a word, fu-past), and reverse time travels towards the *now*. Time, like a double helix DNA model, spirals outwards towards the *fu-past*, or inwards towards the now.

> Sunbeams
> So we dance,
> Spiralling together,
> Tentatively at first,
> Around each other.
> Entwining then,
> Touching, yet
> How can this be?

Helium time is 'timeless' soul time. In descriptions of life between lives, time appears to be equally one second or a million years long, just as deep sleep feels timeless. Here, time cannot be measured, partly because it is not linear. For the purpose of our discussion, the Cabbalah considers sleep to be a small death. So that sleep will transport us into Helium helix time, as we will see later.

Finally, we enter pre-hydrogen time, before the Big Bang. Reverse once again, and here the whole universe is concentrated into one pinpoint of singularity, meaning that the movement of matter, energy and time is from circumference to centre (Figure 18.5). All possible *fu-pasts* and all possible *there-thens* condense into this one point, so that everything exists in potential only.

Here are some examples of Hydrogen time space collapsing into one. (Note, this is Hydrogen, not pre-hydrogen, so they only approximate pre-hydrogen.)

I felt in the presence of a totally pure energy, like meeting God ... realizing all the mistakes of a lifetime ... I feel this unification cleared out lifetimes of symptomatology for me. The joining with this energy was as if a male energy joined with me sexually, but with no desire, pleasure or pain involved.

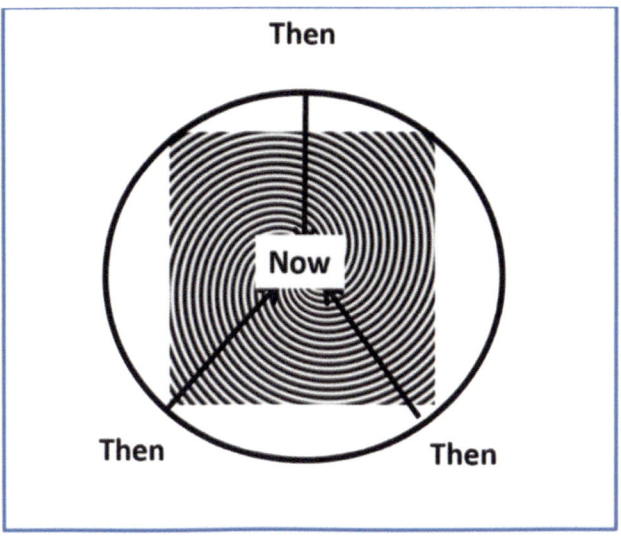

Figure 18.5 *Singularity. Everything is concentrated in the centre, including time*

Let us reverse the sequence, traveling from Big-Bang to Krypton. The Big Bang is an abrupt reversal of direction. Suddenly, rather than collapsing on itself, time-space explodes outwards, from centre to circumference. 'Not-now' becomes time, and 'not-here' becomes space.

Much more one-pointed concentration on whatever I am doing. Not thinking of more than one thing at a time. A lifetime is a very short space of time.

I was having problems assimilating the notion of time; outside time seemed beyond description. I couldn't differentiate between backwards and forwards in time. Felt I had got stuck in time.

Feeling of great release – catharsis – my whole timescale has changed since taking the remedy. Boundaries have disappeared. Lost a lot of boundaries on time.

Soon after, if there is a soon, hydrogen is born, and then helium, with time flowing outwards from centre to circumference, from now to then, in a helical pattern.[8] *Fu-pasts* and *there-thens* begin to manifest on the periphery.

As it incarnates down the spinning labyrinth, the helium soul splits, reverses direction, splits again and enters the body for conception followed by nine months of timeless pregnancy. The helical pattern of this time can be perceived in the formation of a galaxy, the whorl of fingerprints and the crown of an infant (Figures 18.6A,B,C).

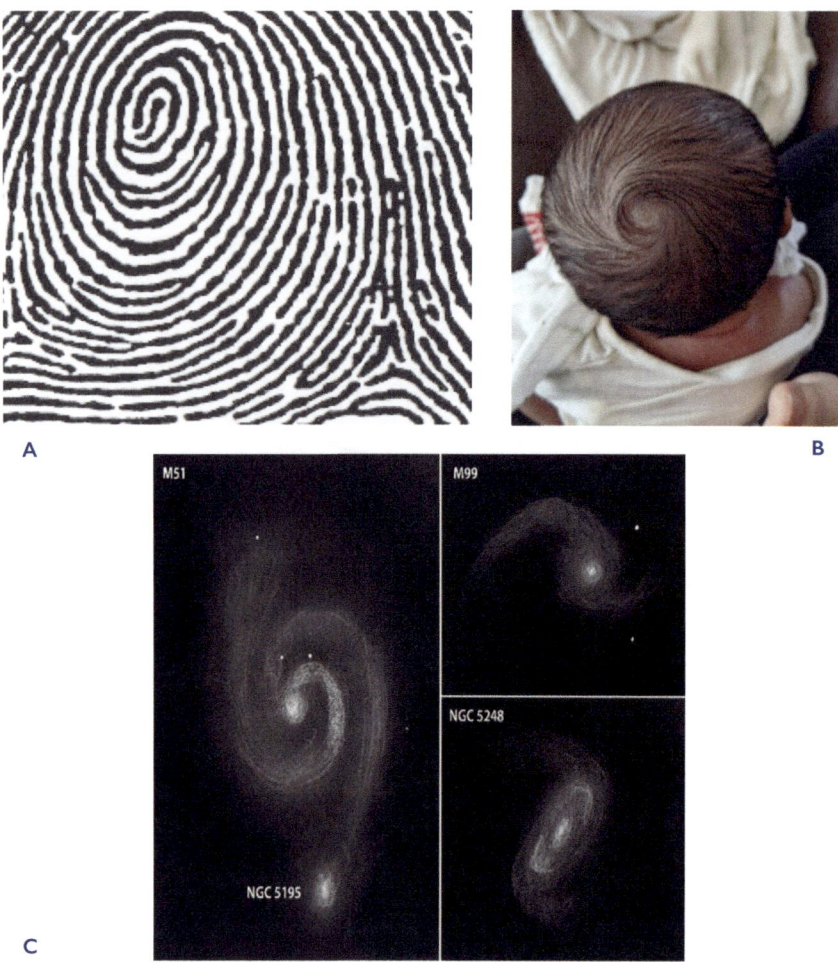

Figure 18.6A,B,C *Time whorls manifesting from Helium into birth*

Finally, a new Neon baby is born into a time corridor.

If Helium represents the pre-Psoric circular time, how did Neon confine this to the Psoric 'arrow of time'? This time-full delusion comes about when we transit from the spiritual Helium soul into the corporal Neon. As described in my Neon book, once the soul enters the body, it divides in two, one half migrating forward to the eyes, the second to the posterior shadow world. It is the front half, observing the world, that confines circular into linear time. Detaching from universal vision, the individual becomes an observer, and the act of observation frames freezes one particular incident of time into a dot. A row of such dots, the continuum of our life, create a line, the Psoric time arrow of Neon. The following are wonderful Neon proving descriptions of this:

I kept seeing the image of a circle, with an arrow going from the top of it, straight up. I was aware of the circle but I could not see the centre of it. My awareness was held on the arrow.

Feel out of control, as if time is moving relentlessly and remorselessly forward, and I'm stuck behind, unable to keep up.

According to quantum physics, time is defined as a fixed event only once it is observed. If unobserved, all possible future-past (fu-past) points become probable realities spread throughout space-time. Thinking of time in this way, it is possible to compare observer-based time (the 'arrow of time') to a river, and observer-less (multidirectional) time to an ocean.

The following is from a paper by scientist and artificial intelligence researcher, Dr. Ben Goertzel:[9]

In quantum physics, it is the observation of a phenomenon that makes the phenomenon definite … Observing a phenomenon makes it 'collapse' from an array of equally real possibilities to one real event, and an array of other 'didn't-happens'.

…. in the microscopic domain everything just exists in a kind of nebulous, atemporal continuum. Then, every once in a while, something becomes observable, and enters the one-dimensional time continuum. The arrow of time does not exist in the universe as a whole. It only exists in individual subjective views of the universe!

… The one direction of time is now viewed as an approximation of the true nature of the universe – an approximation induced by the perceptual limitations of particular observers like us.

In 2013 the physicist Ekaterina Moreva and colleagues[10] working at the National Institute for Research in Optics and Photonics (INRIM) in Turin, confirmed that to a god-like observer outside the universe measuring the evolution of particles, these particles would appear entirely unchanging – and time would not exist. But an internal observer inside the universe would see a difference, which would be a measure of time. Hence time is an emergent phenomenon for 'internal' observers but absent for external ones.[11]

Moving on from Neon, the Argon mirror reverses the direction of the arrow of time once again, so that past is behind and future ahead.

Completing tasks quickly and finally getting things done. Feel I am catching up on lost time and moving on.

And here is what happens when Argon curatively removes this arrow of time delusion:[12,13]

It is as if time didn't exist. And yet, I am functioning. How? I would like more of it. But now I feel that it is completely unmeasured. If it went on much longer, I would become terribly frightened because I remember that a sense of time does exist – that this is not real. (Curative, but too abrupt.)

Onward to Krypton. Time reversal is prominent in the homoeopathic proving of Krypton:

I have the feeling of having time, yet not having time.
I wish I could go backwards in time.
I am the mother of my father and the sister of my husband, and he is my offspring.
Dream that I went to go swimming with a friend's son. The child was in a hurry to incarnate. It was too early because I haven't met the man yet.
Dream of reversal of the seven days.
The River Jordan flowed the other way.

Interestingly, Lord Rayleigh, who discovered krypton, as well as neon, argon and xenon, experimented with reverse time. He postulated that an object traveling faster than the speed of sound while emitting a sound, would result in sound waves that seem to travel in the opposite direction, and so appear to be reversed in time orientation. Recently, Daniele Faccio and team, experimented with Rayleigh's predictions on light waves. By using super-high-speed cameras, they captured a line moving in the opposite direction to the source, as if it had travelled backward in time. The same team used these cameras to 'curve' light, taking pictures around corners (non-line-of-sight (NLOS) imaging).[14]

Krypton, however, has a different take on time reversal. It could not simply flip the direction of the 'arrow of time' once again, that would be so passe. Rather, the Krypton flips inside to out and outside to in, by sending *now* to the periphery, and *then* to the centre (Figure 18.7).

In Krypton, our centre of being becomes the *then-there*, and we are never *here-now*. This is the gateway to chronicity, the root of all pathology. Every rubric in the repertory, every symptom in the materia medica, would be

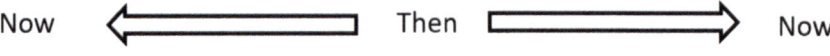

Krypton time

Figure 18.7 Krypton linear pathology. Now then, then here

healthy and appropriate in another *there-then*. For example, salivating when eating is necessary, but salivating during sleep is a problem. Being sympathetic when seeing a hungry, poor man lying in the street is appropriate, but having the same emotion to our abuser would be pathology. As my grandmother said, 'Dirt is only matter in the wrong place'. Pathology is a *fu-past* migrating to the center, while the *here-now*, takes a hike to east of anywhere.

From Krypton:

I've recognised in myself an inability to be here and now. I always work towards some goal 'out there', thus sacrificing the present.

I'm losing it; time is deluding me. Important stuff is becoming unimportant and unimportant things take on great importance and big dimensions.

As if time runs through my fingers. No matter what I do, I can't get a grip of things or time. It just slips through my hands.

When a dose of Krypton is curative of this chronic state of Chronos, the individual returns to original Helium holistic time.

The concept of time has changed. It feels more as a continuum present rather than in compartments of before, past, later, and so forth. (curative)

Very conscious about the present moment, continuum present. (curative)

One of my friends told me about a secret meditation technique which could cut through eons of time and bring you right back to God. (curative)

Until this point, Krypton time still flows in a straight line, but with *then* in the center. Here comes Stage Two. At some stage in the fourth periods development, time curves, becoming circular. So, we are now back to the circular time direction of the first period. However, as opposed to Helium time, *there-then* and *fu-pasts* are in our centre being, while *here-now* move to the periphery (Figure 18.8). And that is how we exist, clinging to yesteryear, clocking in at the office while dreaming of a holiday at the beach, and worrying about the office at the beach. Hence, *The grief history of time!*

You would rightly ask, when does this change from straight time to circular time occur as the fourth period approaches Krypton. I cannot be sure, but my feeling that is in Gallium, as the line is stretched to its max. If you refer back to chapter on the fourth dimension, I discussed this. Here is the Gallium summary on this issue.

Noticing every curve of the terrain. This diagram came up in my head, a circle and a point in the center. Boarding a plane which had to circle around and around. A large circle on the outside. People are sitting in a circle.

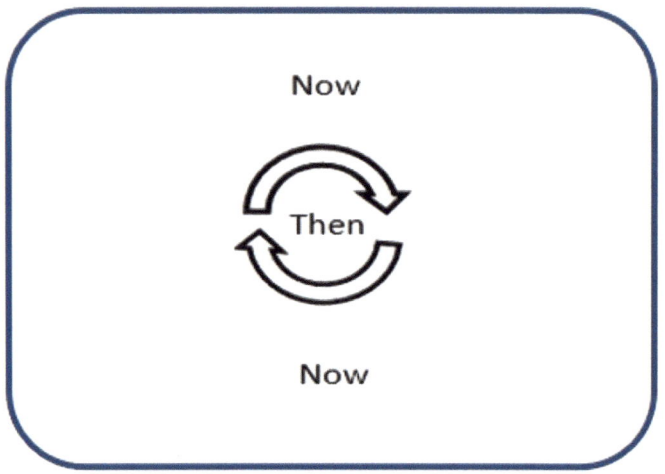

Figure 18.8 *Krypton circular pathology. Round and round, the merry-go-round*

Xenon and Radon will perform some more exciting tricks with the concept of time. But let's give time a break while we go to sleep.

Time as if

Ailments from,
As if.
river never flowed to brook,
nor cloud melt back to sea.
time the great impostor,
frame froze reality.
And throwing her deceptive veil,
defines our every motion,
confining to a notion.
Ailments from,
As if.

History,
As if.
photos in a family album,
groomed chronology,
we dance to rigid rhythm,
we march your one-way street.
Never bending nor reversing,
age to child or tree to seed,
we trek time's linear path,
the sequence of our deeds
History, As if

The miracle of sleep

Clinically, loss of sleep or unrefreshed sleep has been found to be a fore-runner of pathology and even death. Sleep deprivation leads to serious physical and mental disease. Even 60 hours of total sleeplessness results in confusion, loss of memory, lack of coordination, decrease in nerve function, and visual hallucinations.[15] Long-term lack of sleep quickens ageing, increases blood pressure, may lead to diabetes and weight gain, lowers immunity, increases the likelihood of disease and dementia, and leads to premature death.[16] With total sleeplessness, the longest recorded life is 11 days.[17]

In contrast, those with good quality sleep can live long and useful lives. Sleep heals all of these ailments, a true miracle. A person goes to sleep tired at the end of a long day, and awakens refreshed, rejuvenated, and restored, ready for another productive day. With sleep we can live into our 90s and beyond. Sleep is a restorer of life and order, a daily miracle of healing that postpones inevitable decay, disease, and death. Studies suggest that the functions of sleep include recovery of the cellular network, nerve synapses, protein synthesis, metabolic function, endocrine system, energy conservation, emotional stresses and ecological adaptations. Adequate sleep also plays a role in learning, memory and cognitive function, which all deteriorate with sleep deprivation.[15]

To date, science has failed to answer how this process works. There are biological explanations of the physiological processes, but not an essential explanation of what lies behind the sleep phenomenon. According to Mathew Walker, a professor of neuroscience and psychology at the University of California, Berkeley, and author of *Why We Sleep*.[15]

Sleep remains one of the last great biological mysteries. All of the mighty problem-solving methods in science – genetics, molecular biology, and high-powered digital technology – have been unable to unlock the stubborn vault of sleep.

I hope to make a small contribution to this investigation.

Entropy

The law that entropy always increases, holds, I think, the supreme position among the laws of Nature.

Sir Arthur Eddington[18]

The Second Law of Thermodynamics states that the amount of energy within a closed system becomes more and more disordered over time (high entropy).[19] The universe started out in a highly ordered state (low entropy), but with the passing of time, things just get messier and messier. Vegetables rot, cars rust, buildings crumble, stars burn out, our bodies decay. Time hurtles us down a one-way street towards decomposition and death, and there is no way back. The Second Law states that there is a natural tendency of any isolated system to degenerate into a more disordered state. This is so fundamental to physics that it is considered absolute folly to challenge it.

Bio-entropy seems to be accelerated by sleeplessness, in comparison to a life endowed with normal sleep. And while we can enhance life's quality by diet, exercise, or healthy living, these activities require input of energy, which sleep does not. Sleep restores rather than consumes energy. It appears that sleep reverses or at least delays the rapid decay of life, in other words, sleep seems to contradict the second law of thermodynamics, which is unacceptable.

Therefore, I asked myself, how can sleep reverse this process?

After some thought, I arrived at the following conclusion: Sleep does not reverse the second law of thermodynamics. To achieve the miracle of restoration, sleep must reverse time.

Reverse Time

There was a young lady named Bright,
Whose speed was far faster than light;
She started one day
In a relative way,
And returned on the previous night.

H. Reginald Buller[20]

To recap: Time is a relentless one-way path leading towards disorder and death. Sleep reverses this process, reorganising the organism and recharging its battery. Therefore, sleep must be an inverse process to life's wear and tear *over time*. To perform this miracle, *sleep must reverse time*. Certainly, we know that sleep distorts time perception, making a dream's time seem much longer.[16]

The reversal of time is not an unknown concept. Several scientists have proposed theories about particles or information that travel in reverse time.[1] John Gleason Cramer, Jr a professor emeritus of physics at the University of Washington, believes that this reversal of cause and effect provides a basis for non-local effects and entanglement.[21] Bear in mind that *non-local effects and entanglement* are a good description of dreams, where events and places are not related by logic, cause, effect, or proximity. Cramer suggests that every entity in the universe sends out waves both forwards and backwards in time, and that time runs bi-directionally.

In some fields of physics, researchers have proposed the theoretical concept of *retro causality*, in which the 'arrow of time' is reversed so that an effect may happen before a cause.[22] In 2021 a team of physicists has shown how quantum systems can simultaneously evolve along two opposite time arrows – both forward and backward in time.[23] To my mind, these are steps in to understanding the reversal of time, but are either partially correct or irrelevant.

When most people think of time reversal, they imagine time traveling backwards along the same path as it travelled forward, i.e., from present to past, as in 'Back to the Future' movies. This would be a delusion. If a glass of wine the falls and shatters on the floor, we imagine that time reversal will cause it to magically reassemble itself into a shiny, new glass of Merlot. Sadly, this is not going to happen.

Loschmidt's Paradox states that a shattered glass will not become whole again even if time reverses, and an egg will not unscramble itself back into its shell.[24] This misunderstanding is a result of imagining time to be travelling in a straight arrow from past to future, which, as we have already seen, is a Psoric delusion. Time presents in this form only as it is frame-frozen in the minds of those observing it.

Ben Goertzel, the computer scientist and artificial intelligence researcher mentioned earlier, states:[9]

> This time-reversibility of our physical equations is not a mathematical fluke; it is a scientific fact that reflects a deep philosophical truth. It reflects the truth that unidirectional time is not fundamental. Unidirectional time is here, but it emerges from a more fundamental substrate of bidirectional (or perhaps even multidirectional) time.

Thus, the reversal of time is a distinct possibility. But not a reversal along a future/past 'arrow of time'. That would be naïve and simplistic.

---

[1] For further study, see Clopton RW. Introducing the Space Time Helix and the Possible Destruction of All Matter. *Space Intelligence.com*. Available online at: http://tinyurl.com/mwzyr66e

If we return to the concepts I explained in *A Grief History of Time* above, we can think of time reversal in a totally new way, by imposing it onto the helical time model of the first period. This means that during waking hours, time flows from a central point of now to a multitude of *fu-pasts*. During sleep, time reverses its direction of flow from the *fu-pasts* towards a central point of *now*. Reverse time *does* not flow towards the past. It flows towards the *now*. And from a homoeopathic perspective, this is the direction of health. My Law of Cure states: 'The direction of cure is towards the here and now.[25] So, let us make a quick detour to examine some common denominators of sleep and homoeopathic cures.

Sleep and homoeopathy

Sleep and homoeopathic healing echo each other. Sleep is a miracle, just like homoeopathy. After sleep and after a good remedy we are restored, renewed, and refreshed, with many of our ailments and stresses healed. One of the best results of a good remedy is an improvement in sleep quality.

Both homoeopathy and sleep reverse time from the *fu-pasts* to the *here and now*; hence both are curative. After a good remedy, when we are more centred in the *now*, we have the freedom to let go of long past traumas, just as sleep and dreams may help us address, resolve, and forget past issues.

On the other hand, unrefreshing, insufficient or untimely sleep fails to perform the daily miracle of restoring health. Hahnemann's objection to coffee may have been its capacity to withdraw energy deposits from the depth of people's being (adrenals), allowing them to charge their day, while robbing their sleep of its miraculous refreshing qualities by causing superficial, restless sleep.

While similar remedies restore us to the *here and now*, provings, which are dissimilar remedies, take their provers towards any one of the infinite *there-thens* in the *fu-past*, a journey into the sea of probabilities and the infinite variety of possible disease forms (states not appropriate to our terrestrial *here and now*). Provings morph us into crusaders, space pilots or Neanderthals, and these ideas repeat throughout the proving. Provers' dreams take on repetitive patterns according to the genus of the remedy, the reflection of being stuck in another time and place. This is different from the random dreams of heathy people.

Understanding the directions of flow of time might shed some light on the difference between Hering's Law of Cure and mine. In Hering's Law *symptoms* travel from centre to periphery as cure evolves. But this is a daytime logic, unravelling from now to the countless *fu-pasts*. (Note that while old symptoms return to the past, aggravations accelerate into the future.) My law of cure is night-time logic; the reason symptoms are escaping to the periphery, is that the soul is returning to the *here and now*.

Finally, the *Tao te Ching* states

> *In the pursuit of learning, every day something is acquired.*
> *In the pursuit of Tao, every day something is dropped.*
> *Less and less is done*
> *Until non-action is achieved.*
> *When nothing is done, nothing is left undone.*

Lao Tzu[26]

The pursuit of learning happens during waking hours. During the day we run around, acquiring, learning and expanding energy. During the night we let go, doing less and less, as we forget, heal and gain energy. We forget we slept, we forget our dreams as they dissolve into the night, we forget to run around holding our breath. This is similar to homoeopathy. After receiving a good remedy, we forget we had all those troublesome symptoms. Patients often forget they ever had homoeopathy. And they forget to pay. These are all well-known phenomena.

To examine a possible connection between forgetting and time reversal, we will visit Lorenzo Maconne.

The second law reversed – Maccone's proposal

> *Composers make; decomposers unmake. And unless decomposers unmake,*
> *there isn't anything that composers can make with.*

Merlin Sheldrake[27]

Theoretical physicist Maccone provides a novel explanation of the nature of entropy, that sheds new light on my hypothesis regarding sleep and dreams. Maccone suggests that entropy can in fact decrease, but it is impossible to detect this process because it leaves no trace of information in its wake.[28]

When entropy increases, as in the decaying universe apparent to mankind, there is always a trail of information left behind, which we call history. According to Maccone, however, when entropy decreases there is no record of anything having happened. Memory and data are simply sucked up, and since there is no evidence, it seems that the reversing phenomena never happened. Physics cannot study processes where entropy has decreased, due to a complete absence of information. This solution allows for time-reversing, in agreement with the laws of physics; but it is not observable, in agreement with the Second Law of Thermodynamics.

By examining Maccone's idea in relation to helical time, the only way information and memory can vanish during the reverse flow of time, is if reverse time flows towards the *now*, rather than towards the past. Thus, forward time creates a *fu-past* trail of information. Reverse-time, however, evaporates all traces of information, because in the now, all past and futures are lost. History and information fold into a single moment where they cease to exist. In the singular *here and now*, there is nothing to calculate, forecast, consider or remember. Everything is in order. Which is why we meditate.

And so, the word 'reverse' may not be accurate. Rather than reverse, I will now say 'restore time', meaning restore to the *here and now*. This is the word Hahnemann uses in Paragraph One, and for good reason. The common Psoric fallacy is that by restoring the sick to health, like restoring an old chair to its former glory, Hahnemann meant we go back to childhood, conception or Neandertal. Not so. Restoring the sick to health means to restore them to the *here and now*. *The direction of cure is a movement towards the 'here and now'.*

If we return to our sleep model, during waking hours, time flows from centre to periphery, from the *now* towards the *fu-past*. According to the Second Law of Thermodynamics, this direction of time increases entropy or chaos, and hurtles humanity towards disease and death. During sleep however, time reversal restores time from the *fu-past* towards the *now* – from chaos to organisation. Sleep, just like the action of homoeopathic remedies, is curative, restores health, order and rejuvenates life by spiralling from *then-there* towards the *here-now*. Actually, at this point both time and space are one.

Dream time

> *If I had a world of my own, everything would be nonsense. Nothing would be what it is, because everything would be what it isn't. And contrary wise, what is, it wouldn't be. And what it wouldn't be, it would. You see?*
>
> Lewis Carroll[29]

How does the phenomenon of time reversal (then to now) manifest in our dreams?

While time does progress during sleep on the material level (organs, and biological processes), sleep reverses the direction of flow of our inner consciousness and vital force, causing time and logic to flow backwards. Eddington, who developed the concept of the '*arrow of time*', states that its reversal would render the external world nonsensical.[30] This would mean that the logical progression of daytime logic or *common-sense*, would turn into *non-sense* when time reverses, which I have postulated happens during sleep. Because, as we know, most dreams are nonsensical.

Logic helps us organise our day and keep it in order, but this requires energy. Logic is our attempt to stop or at least slow down entropy. Logically we know we have to visit the dentist, do the shopping and cook. Reversing the direction of time at night means inverting logic into un-logic. In the dream world, logic itself flows backwards, creating non-sense. Nonsensical dreams are therefore an indicator of the reversal of logic as well as time during sleep. Other terms that describe non-logical phenomenon are 'magic' or 'miracle'. As in a Harry Potter book, during dreams, the dreamer can shrink, fly, breathe under water, or visit other planets. In dreams, the dreamer witnesses magic, both good and bad. Magic parallels the miracle of sleep as a non-sensical reverser of entropy and restorer of health. The magical world of dreams acts as a counterbalance to daily logic. In dreams, the 'logical world' of Krypton can jump back through the mirror into the magical Argon dream world of childhood, Neverland, while reversing time flow from entropy into organisation and rejuvenating our youth.[31]

In another parallel between dreams and homoeopathy, Samuel Hahnemann, emphasises the importance of strange, rare and peculiar symptoms as the best tool to finding the remedy[32] a counter-balance to common logical symptoms. Nonsense, miracles and magic fall into the category of 'Strange Rare and Peculiar' (SRP). Both dreams and SRPs give insight to the inner, non-logical, magical person.

Dreams take us to strange, rare and peculiar places, far from the *here and now*. During dreams we visit the countless *fu-past* possibilities. One might say that during sleep the observer vanishes, thus allowing our consciousness to surf on helical time and allowing the possibility of all possibilities.

Relating Maccone's suggestion to dreams, most of the time people cannot recall dreams because dreams are a result of sleep's reversal of time from high entropy decay towards low entropy order. As an organism reorganises itself during sleep, the trail of information is simply swallowed up. Therefore, sleep or dreams cannot be recalled, but instead simply dissolve on awakening. And while you might protest and say you do remember dreams, these are only a small percent of what you dreamt. According to scientists, we forget up to 95% of all dreams shortly after waking.[33] "There is much more dreaming going on than we remember," says Tore Nielsen at the University of Montreal, Canada. "It's hours and hours of mental experiences and we remember a few minutes."[34] Most dreams are recalled only if people are woken during REM sleep, make an effort to remember them, or if the dreams are *patho-logical*. Otherwise, most people remember a dream one or twice a week, probably one out of many.

While dreams are extremely difficult to study, there is anecdotal evidence to support my theory. Some systems of psychoanalysis interpret dream sequences in reverse order, and there are certain dreams that can only be understood by unravelling them backwards in time. People often recall their dreams from back to front, and during dreams they sometimes *know* what will happen next, scene by scene. The experience can be described like walking towards the rear of a forward-moving train. There is a sense of déjà vu, because the scene was observed previously in the dream, and its movement is backwards through time.

Furthermore, the dreamer can change the past in their dreams. If the dreamer encounters a scene in a dream that is illogical or inconvenient, they can decide to change it into something more suitable. Additionally, revisiting the same scene later in the dream, the dreamer may see that it has magically changed.

For instance, I dreamed of a patient that came to my home. My wife went to get the requested medication and came back naked, which felt inappropriate. The next moment I reversed the sequence, and my wife appeared dressed. I simply rearranged events to suit what I wanted, going back in time and changing things that did not fit.

Some people have clairvoyant dreams, because when time reverses, it becomes possible to *remember the future*. In his article, *The Physics of Now*, physicist James B. Hartle[35] postulates that remembering the future is within the possibility of fourth dimension space-time. Hence, it is possible to travel backwards in time from future to past, at least during sleep.

I believe that dreams that are logical, repetitive, and common rather than strange, rare, and peculiar are an echo of pathology, a rational obstacle to the miracle of sleep. Recurring dreams form logical patterns that are amenable to analysis. A healthy person's dreams cannot and, for the most part, should not be interpreted; these dreams belong to the world of *non-sense*. Dream analysis should be limited to *patho-logical* dreams, where the organism is crying for help. Here, echoes of a person's pathology infect the person's magical world of dreams with logical patterns that can be traced, tracked and interpreted. Otherwise, we are invading non-logical night with our logical day. Even 'problem-solving' dreams, such as Mendeleev decoding the pattern of the periodic table, reflect a problem unsolved. Likewise, I believe that excessive lucid dreaming is an attempt to control that which should be left uncontrolled, the force of logical day time invading the night's magic. When it comes to healthy non logical dreams, forget them, and do not try to make or put sense into them. On the other hand, daydreams, insanity, delirium, drug-induced states, or feelings of déjà vu are the invasion of the magical world of dreams by the daily world of reason.

It is interesting that Christopher Nolan, the director of the film *Inception*,[36] also directed *Me Inception* deals with people penetrating the world of dreams as a form of industrial espionage. *Memento* follows the journey of an amnesiac backwards along a shattered memory lane. Using various triggers, he travels back through time in reverse order, chunk by chunk. This is very similar to the way that dreams are remembered. Nolan also directed *Insomnia*,[37] depicting the effects of loss of sleep, and *Following*,[38] where the chronological order of events is jumbled. The correlations with reverse time creating non-sensical sequences during dreams are obvious.

Time opposite mind

From a relativity point of view, consciousness or mind flows in the opposite direction of time, just as the station seems to travel in an opposite direction to a moving train. In health, the mind balances the deterioration resulting from the passage of time by moving in the opposite direction; during the day, when time flows towards the peripheral *fu-past*, the healthy consciousness mind streams towards the central *now*. Because the flow of time to the periphery causes chaos, human consciousness balances this with an inner order.

On the other hand, during sleeping hours, time flows inward towards the central axis of *here and now*, unravelling the destructive consequences of wake-time. Dreams stemming from the unconscious mind flow in the opposite direction, towards the peripheral *fu-past*, the infinity of diverse times and places of the dream world (Figures 18.9 and 18.10).

The above occurs in a state of health. However in disease (i.e., Psora) this process reverses itself. Polarities flip and the flow of time reverses. Hence, during pathological sleep, instead of moving towards the *here and now*, time flows towards the *fu-past* and is unrestorative and unrefreshing. Dreams, moving in the opposite direction are of the *here and now*, recreating events of the day, or logical patterns which are constantly recurring daytime issues of the dreamer.

Conversely, waking time in disease spirals towards the *here-now*, the egocentric existence, rather than to the *fu-past*. At the same time, the conscious mind wanders off towards the *fu-past*, down memory lane, and along future pathways. People dwell on the past, worry about tomorrow, and prefer the neighbour's green grass. This is termed *dis-position*: out of central position. In disease, the flow of time and mind in Figures 18.9 and 18.10 are reversed.

The reader may wonder why awake-time spiralling towards the now in disease does not restore an individual, since it seems to be moving away from entropy. This is because the universe is expanding towards random

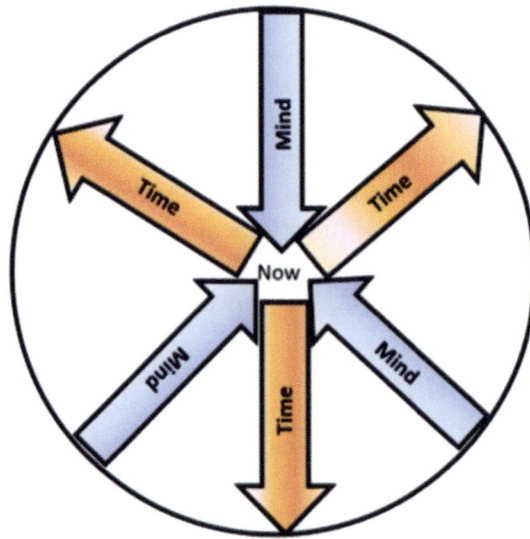

Figure 18.9 *In health, while awake, time flows to the periphery and entropy. Mind flows towards now to maintain balance*

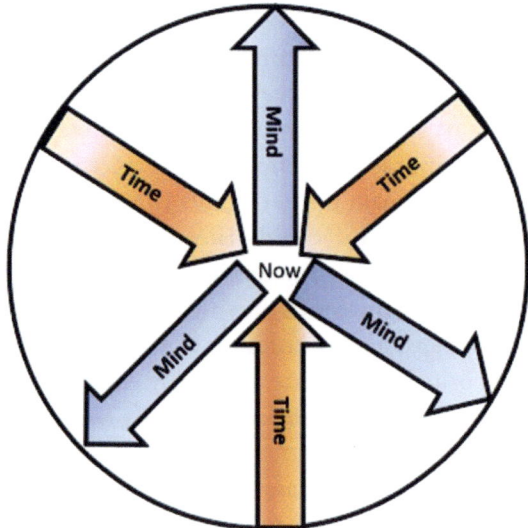

Figure 18.10 *In health, while asleep, time flows to the now and restoration. The unconscious mind flows towards the fu-past (dreams)*

chaos and ultimate destruction. To counteract this, people expend an enormous amount of energy trying to cling to life, to stop or delay the inevitable decaying process. Each person strives vainly to organise her world, but this is like trying to stop a river flowing into the sea. The end results are control and perfectionism, the most common pathologies of the 21st Century, and their opposing chaotic cancers. Ultimately, in disease, sleep is not refreshing and daytime is experienced as exhausting.

Types of dreams

Here we are all, by day; by night we're hurl'd
By dreams, each one into a several world.

Robert Herrick[39]

Based on the concept explained above, we can categorise two extreme types of dreams, with many shades of grey in between. From these we may construct a hierarchy of dreams in relation to heath and illness.

On one extreme are random, crazy, and nonsensical dreams, which indicate a reversed flow of time and logic, and are therefore a function of healthy sleep. These dreams act as a window to the magical strange, rare and peculiar – a world that restores the human organism's deterioration. Here magic antidotes logic.

On the other extreme are logical, sequential, or repetitive dreams, such as dreams of the day's events. These indicate a normal day-time flow from past to future. Since sleep should reverse the flow of time and logic to restore well-being, this order is unhealthy. Failing to convert normal day-time logic into sleep's 'reverse time' is a problematic sign that leads to chronic disease, entropy, and death. If one spends 10 hours a day in the office and another six in dream time office, that cannot be a harmonious health.

Between these two extremes are many shades of grey, dreams which are part random and part logical. For example, a person might dream of unsuccessful efforts to fly. The flying reflects magic, while the unsuccessful part reflects an inner pathology, an echo of stuck emotional states such as failure to succeed in business or in love. Hence, these dreams are easy to analyse.

From a homoeopathic point of view, one-off nonsense dreams are insignificant. Patients may say something like: 'Last night I dreamt of a purple dolphin wearing a necklace.' However, this dream only occurred once, hence it is of little interest in finding a remedy, unless they happen to have anything dolphin or purple in their case, e.g purple fingernails. If we reverse this idea into the logical day world, would you repertorise the following symptom: 'I brushed my teeth this morning'? No, because it is common, logical and repetitive, the opposite of the SRP dream. Hence the following:

Sherr's Law of Values of Dreams

- Common symptoms have low value.
- SRP symptoms have high value.
- Common dreams have high value.
- SRP dreams have low value.

From this we can construct my Hierarchy of Dreams, from most pathological to healthiest:

- Repeating bad dreams.
- Repeating OK/good dreams.
- No dreams.
- Random bad dreams.
- Random good dreams.
- Discombobulated dreams (see next section: Where and When are Dreams).

So, if a person is experiencing recurring dreams of a childhood trauma, and following a remedy they have recurring dreams of a nice experience, that is positive. But if they progress from random bad dreams to recurring bad dreams, that would be a negative direction, because logic (repetition/pattern) has invaded the night.

Note that proving dreams, even if SRPs, are significant, because the proving pushes all provers into one particular corner of the 'sea of all possibilities'. One prover may dream of a necklace, another of a dolphin, and another of a dolphin wearing a necklace. All the provers are traveling toward the same corner of the multiverse.

Where and when are dreams

We have established that dreams occur in the infinite world of possible *fu-pasts and there-thens*. Dreams take us to the strangest of places and far exceed our imagination. I remember a particular dream I once had: a world with a wooden sun and beings that looked like giant chess pieces. Where is this land? Does it exist in some other reality, dimension, or time in the *fu-past*? Has anyone else ever visited it in their dreams? Perhaps dreams are amalgamated scraps of collective consciousness or travels across the multiverse.

Certainly dreams can go back to the long past, to worlds of dinosaurs and crusaders, or to the future, predicting events yet to come. They can take their dreamers to strange and unknown locations. Perhaps they indicate another being's reality, or a mix of many realities. Perhaps they are the combination of all experiences everywhere, a voyage into the *sea of all possibilities* into which people tune, just as a TV set picks up a variety of broadcasts. This would be akin to visiting the 7th, 8th, and 9th dimensions. Dreams take us far into the collective experience.

Analysing the strange, rare, and peculiar dreams of a healthy person, therefore, is a bit like analysing the soul next door, on the next planet, or in the next millennium. There is no logical connection to one's life pattern. The homoeopath should be aware of these dreams, yet not dwell on them. In disease, however, the slowed down and restricted spin of the vital force is not fast enough to disperse most individuals' soul fragments up to these collective levels, and so dreams remain in the personal domain, reflecting the repetitive pattern of each individual's pathology.

Yet dreams also have a locality. I have often found that when sleeping in someone else's bed or in a new environment, that my dreams may take on a hint of the owner's or the location's dreams. I once visited Zanzibar on a romantic holiday with my wife. At the time she knew nothing of its wretched history as a slave station. Yet all night she dreamt of slaves being chained together and sent away to sea, never to see their families again. She awoke shocked and crying. Hence, dreams are also a local TV station that dreamers can tune into when they are near.

In the previous section I mentioned discombobulated dreams. By this I mean dreams where identities morph. Your uncle becomes your sister, and your sister turns into yourself. I place these healthiest in the hierarchy as, apart from being extremely non-sensical, they echo the transformation of soul fragments mixing, which occurs during death, as described in my Helium book. As death is the ultimate helical time moving towards the *here and now*, this would afford the most replenishing sleep.

During sleep, as the vital force spins in reverse, the soul uncoils into primary soul fragments.[ii] These soul fragments disperse as they travel high up into the universal vortex, known as Akashic records,[iii] simple substance (Kent's Swedenborgian term for Akashic records), or collective uncon-sciousness. Here they mix with other universal soul fragments from the collective sea of souls. The faster an individual's 'reverse' spin, the further into the collective they disperse. Fragments of souls and of various locations coalesce into an entangled non-logical mix. Hence, the healthiest dreams belong to the public domain rather than to individual persona. The

---

[ii] For a fuller explanation of soul fragment, see Sherr J. *The Dynamic Materia Medica of the Noble Gases: Helium*, Glasgow: Saltire Books, 2013.

[iii] Akashic records (Akasha is a Sanskrit word meaning, 'sky, space or aether, are collectively understood to be a collection of mystical knowledge that is encoded in the aether; i.e., on a non-physical plane of existence. See *Crystalinks*, http://www. crystalinks.com/

Jewish canons called these *Dreams of Spain*: a man sleeps in Israel and dreams of Spain – meaning a non-local effect. During actual sleep, the Zohar explains, 59 of the 60 parts of our soul leave our bodies, leaving only 1/60 to sustain us physically.[40]

Dreams are a cosmic soup in which all possibilities and probabilities mix. In dreams, reality as the dreamer perceives it disintegrates into atoms and molecules of people, places, times and natural phenomena to reform into an endless variety of permutations. Grandmothers, rocket ships, snakes, childhood friends, oceans, stars and crocodiles fuse to create an impossible movie in which the director has lost the plot, cut all the clips into shreds, mixed them on the floor and randomly spliced them together.

Helix and Gyre

> *Turning and turning in the widening gyre*
> *The falcon cannot hear the falconer;*
> *Things fall apart; the centre cannot hold;*
> *Mere anarchy is loosed upon the world,*
> *The blood-dimmed tide is loosed, and everywhere*
> *The ceremony of innocence is drowned;*
>
> W.B. Yeats[41]

The helix, a three-dimensional spiral, represents the dynamic pattern of universal and vital motion. The footprint of this motion is evident in many natural and biological structures: the spiral-shaped patterns of hair on the human crown, of fingerprints, and in the double helix of DNA. Blood swirls as it rushes through arteries, which are designed with a helical twist to encourage this whirling flow. An ovum rotates when a sperm approaches it. There are beautiful, logarithmic spiral patterns in flowers, claws, horns, teeth, snails and plants. Oceans circulate in gyres and galaxies spiral. Remarkably, there is at least one galaxy which seems to be in the shape of a double helix.[42]

As discussed earlier, time flows in a helical pattern, just like the universal vital force. Hence, it relates directly to the vital force. In fact, it is possible to say that the vital force *is* time: a series of rotating neuro-hormonal clocks that synchronise with the universe.[43]

The double helix was described by poet, writer and philosopher, William Butler Yeats, who describes the motion of our inner being:

> The mind, whether expressed in history or in the individual life, has a precise movement, which can be quickened or slackened but cannot be fundamentally altered, and this movement can be expressed by a mathematical form, and this form is the gyre.[44] (Figure 18.12)

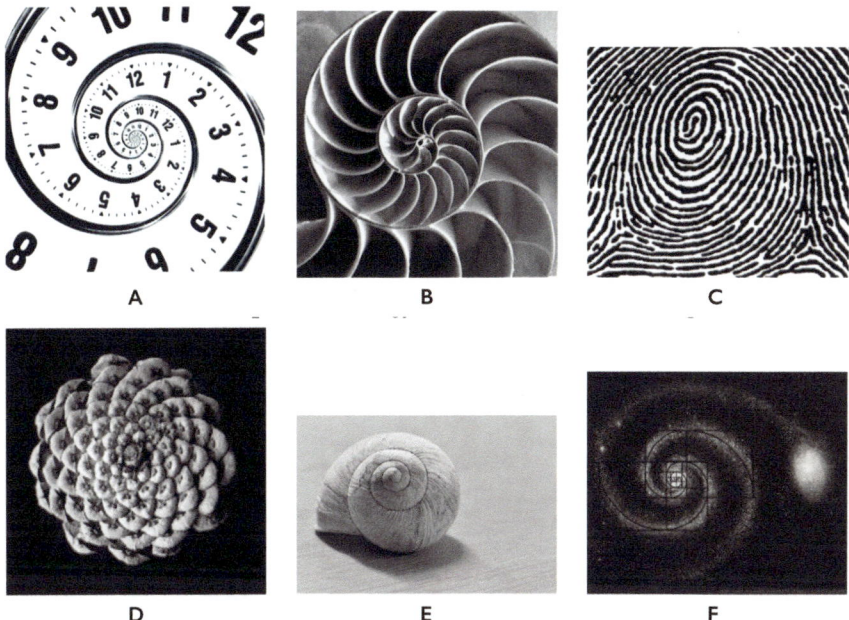

Figure 18.11.A-F Helix, the dynamic pattern of universal and vital motion

in a progressively wider spiral while time adds another dimension, creating the form of a helix or funnel vortex. Once the gyre reaches its point of maximum expansion it begins to narrow until it reaches an endpoint, which is the origin of a new gyre'.[45]

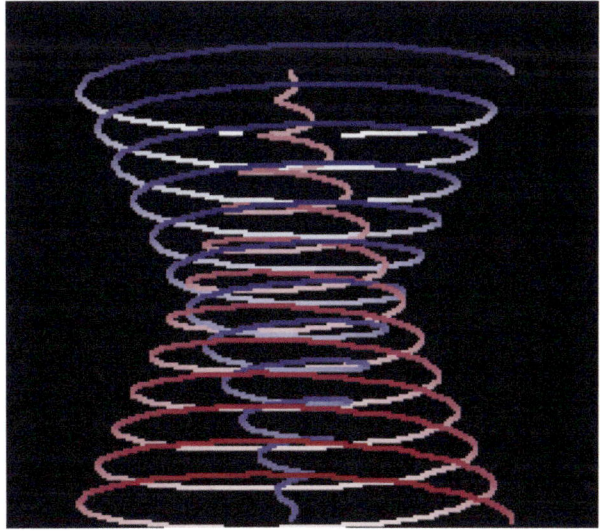

Figure 18.12 A gyre as described by William Butler Yeats

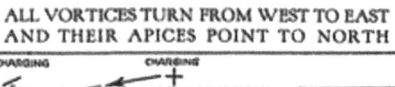

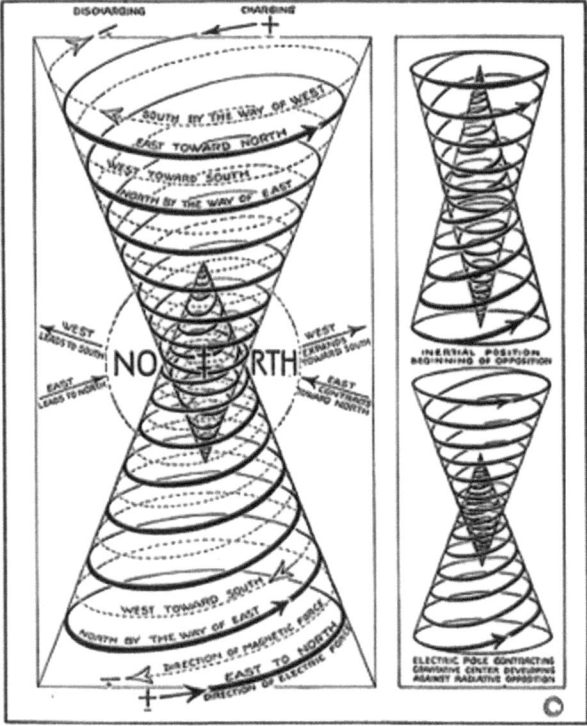

MASS IS ACCUMULATED AROUND A VORTEX.   A VORTEX IS FORMED BY THE CON-
TRACTION OF THE AXIS OF TWO OPPOSING CONES OF ENERGY. THE GREATER THE
CONTRACTION THE GREATER THE ACCELERATION OF MOTION WITHIN THE VORTEX.

Figure 18.13 Vortex

Walter Russell, well known philosopher, painter, sculptor, and author, also envisioned the double-coil helix as the basic pattern of the universe, and used it as a template to design a powerful generator (Figure 18.13).[46]

The double helix represents two coils entwined within each other. When an electric coil (like that in a dynamo) revolves in a magnetic field, it creates electricity (Figure 18.14). When an electric current flows through a coil it creates a magnetic field; and when two electric coils are in proximity (as in a transformer), they cause an *induction*, creating and transferring an electromagnetic field. Based on these principles, the human, revolving, vital, double helix creates a biodynamic life force.[47]

Based on the universal patterns discussed above, it makes sense that the vital force is in fact two spirals flowing in opposite directions. The reason the vital force spirals is that it must oppose external forces in order to survive. These inimical forces may come from any direction: viruses, cold wind, excessive sun, spoilt food, angry bosses, solar radiation, or the

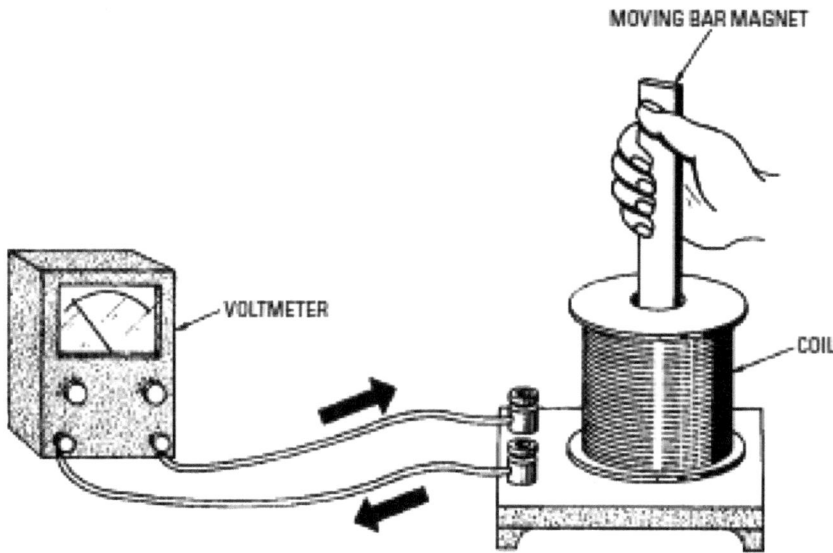

Figure 18.14 *An electric coil revolving in a magnetic field creates electricity*

magnetic fields of the earth. By spinning, the vital force creates a centri-fugal force that can repel these invaders. Like a revolving Tai Chi master, the vital force must be capable of facing any direction at any given moment. It must adapt to change, and therefore it must be capable of change.

If the vital force spins, how fast would this spinning be? Because the maximum speed of external change is the speed of light, the vital force must match it by spinning at or near the speed of light. Truly, human beings are beings of light. Recent discoveries have shown that the human body literally glows, emitting a visible light in extremely small quantities at levels that rise and fall during the day.[48]

Based on these ideas, the vital force is composed of spiralling light. Perhaps this light beam is just a carrier, and the soul that inhabits it lends this light its unique characteristics by modulating it, just as speech modulates a carrier radio wave.

From the proving of Helium, I have learned that the helical motion of the vital force is the result of the soul passing through a spiral maze during reincarnation, leaving helical patterns in its wake.[49]

In inner vision, seeing the shape of a maze. A spiral maze. The spiral of the self and the search for self, symbolising the wandering of the soul circling inward and outward.

Then I have an image of spiralling downwards through lilac and mauves and white vibrations, and as I do, I pass through many flashes of other lives and experiences that I am simultaneously living and passing through to get to this point of birth, this point of incarnation. And here I will stop for a 'time', and how illusory is time?! before I pass onwards in my soul's journey.

As the universal energy swirls through the vortex of archetypes, the helix it leaves in its wake crystallises into material shapes and forms. This vortex is the gateway between the invisible formative world and its material mirror image. Like water rotating through a funnel, the soul's journey through the cosmic labyrinth spins into a life force, acquiring and remembering the rotating shape of its formative vessel. Some palm readers claim that the soul's revolving pattern is reflected in the spiral thumb print, indicating its life mission.[50]

The revolving vital force can be compared to a gyroscope.[51] As a gyroscope spins, it remains upright even if the object upon which it stands is. Because of its spin, the gyroscope resists the external forces that operate on it. Like a healthy person, the gyroscope defies gravity. Defying gravity literally means defying the grave.

When the human vital gyroscope is fresh from the vortex of the soul's descent and spinning at or near the speed of light, the individual is capable of remaining upright in spite of life's tilts, thus repelling most attacks on its organism. However, as the human vital gyroscope slows down due to the friction of terrestrial existence, it loses the power to resist gravity and other external forces. Once it begins to wobble and becomes unstable, chronic sickness and old age develop (Figure 18.15). If an individual's vital gyroscope stops spinning, the person dies.

To rejuvenate one's spin and regain life's vital power, the gyroscope must be rewound in the opposite direction. It is for this reason that many *life-prolonging* exercises such as Sufidervish whirling or the Five Tibetan Rites involve spinning.

As mentioned, sleep is the greatest life rejuvenator due to its time reversal mechanism. Sleep is a rewinding of our vital gyroscope in the opposite direction to that of daily life. During sleep, the human vital force rotates in reverse spin, re-coiling each person's life.

Here are some more Helium symptoms describing this process:

No sleep, no leaving the body, no reprieve, ever more inwards, but it felt I needed to persevere and reverse the process.

Dream: Recognising when people were unwell by the fact that they walked backwards.

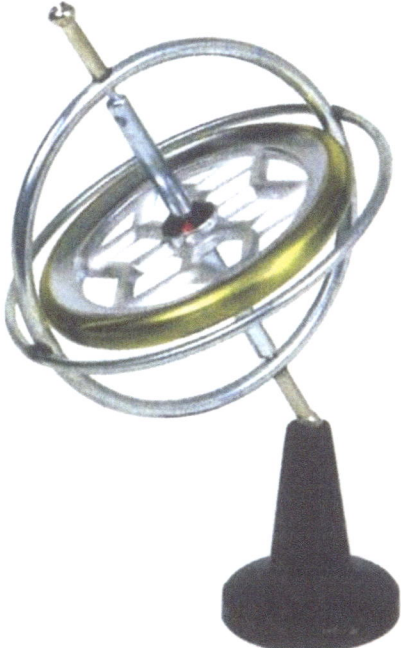

Figure 18.15 *Gyroscope*

Finally, it is now clear why children, and more so teenagers, need many hours of sleep. The young ones' vital gyroscopes spin much faster and longer, and therefore need more rewinding. I am not sure this is fair, but it is the nature of the game.

It is for this reason children also need more play, a magical world that antidotes the grim adult logic.

Reversing the Gyre

The vital gyroscope spins at or near the speed of light. Sleep reverses the direction of the vital gyroscope. However, it does not make sense that the vital force, before reversing into sleep, will slow down from the speed of light to zero, and then start revolving in the opposite direction, accelerating back to the speed of light. If that were the case, people might rapidly grow old and die just before falling asleep. There has to be another mechanism in which the vital force does not slow down but simply reverses direction.

I believe that the solution lies in the double helix or gyre pattern. Both coils, one inside the other, spiral in opposite directions. Each is a light wave carrier modulated by the soul's unique pattern. During wake time,

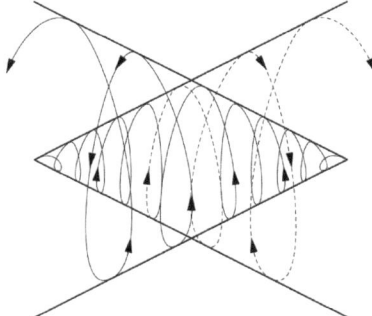

Figure 18.16 *The double gyre of time, flowing both ways. Human consciousness can alternate between the two directions from wake to sleep time*

consciousness or soul modulation is on one coil. But during sleep, this modulation transfers by induction to the counter spinning coil, thus changing direction fairly quickly and without slowing down. Basically, this is a simple reversal of polarities, rather than a change of direction.

According to these thoughts, it is not really a reversal of direction that occurs when individuals switch from wake to sleep and vice versa, but rather a flip of consciousness from one spiral of the gyre to the other, each flowing in a different direction (Figures 18.16 and 18.17).

This moment of change between the coils, or the reversal of polarities, is crucial and delicate. This is the gateway between the worlds of logic and magic where one may pass through the mirror to the other side. Some

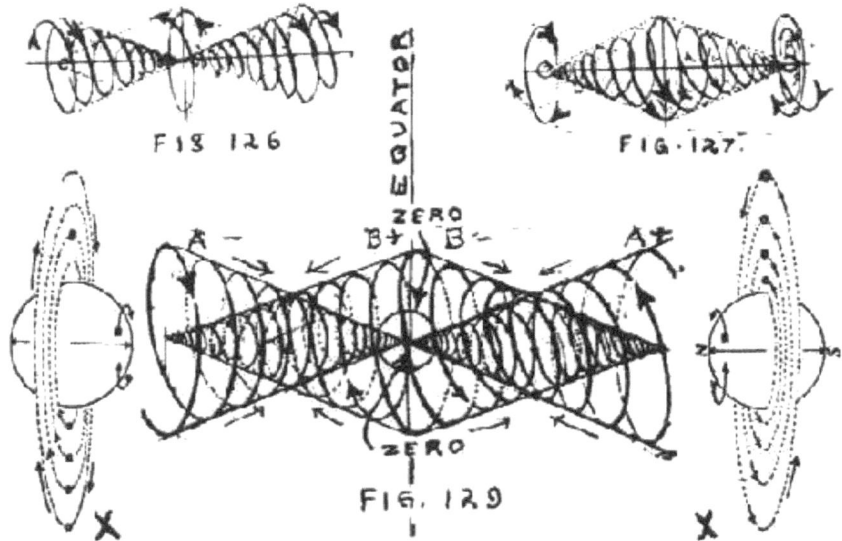

Figure 18.17 *Double coils with reverse flow*

remedy pictures display a weakness at this point, which might show for instance as jerking or twitching on falling asleep, a result of a faulty electric *changeover*. As an example, let us look at Argentum metallicum, well known for shocks and jerks on falling asleep.

Argentum metallicum is also one of the main remedies for difficulty falling asleep, disturbed and unrefreshed sleep – the inability to reverse polarities into refreshing sleep leads to a rapid decay into old age. J.T. Kent says about this about Argentum metallicum: '... he is really a wreck, an old broken-down constitution when he is yet young. A man of forty is like one of eighty.'[52]

Note that this reverse of polarity and electrical flow from daytime to sleep time is essentially the same as the electrical charge crossover that occurs during orgasm, that of electrical tension and relaxation.[iv]

Summary

Sleep reverses decay. In fact, it is the most curative of all medicines. Time hurtles us towards degeneration, in accordance with the incontrovertible Second Law of Thermodynamics. Therefore, the only way sleep can reverse this process is by the reversal of time. However, this is not a simplistic reversal from future to past along an 'arrow of time'. Sleep transports us to a dimension where there is no observer, and consequently time is transformed outside of the terrestrial 'arrow of time' to the more spiritual helical time. Instead of time reversal traveling back to the past, it travels from a myriad of *fu-pasts* towards the *here and now*. Sleep, homoeopathy, and meditation refresh our being and restore health by centring us in the dynamic *now*. According to philosophical and scientific sources, this direction of time leads to forgetting there was a history.

During time reversal, the logical energy we use to slow down decay crumbles, as it is not needed. Dreams represent this by being non-sensical, reverse-logic, strange, peculiar, and magical. And the more non-sensical they are, the healthier the dream.

In a healthy state, during waking hours, time flows from centre to periphery, and mind or consciousness from the periphery towards the *here and now*. Entropy or decay ensue, and people progress towards death. This would happen a lot faster if not for the reverse process of sleep.

During healthy sleep, time flows towards the *here and now*, towards low entropy and high organization. Thus, sleep is restorative. It rewinds our

---

iv For more on this idea one should study Wilhelm Reich. *Der Orgasmus als Elektrophysiologische Entladung*. (The Orgasm as an Electrophysiological Discharge). Available online at: http://tinyurl.com/3wht28uy

vital gyroscope. When our centre being travels towards the *here-now*, dreams travel to the *there-thens* chaotic array of random possibilities.

Because time's direction of flow during sleep is towards the *now*, it leaves no trace and is undetectable. Thus, people normally cannot remember sleep, but they wake refreshed and with renewed vigour and health.

In illness, waking time flows from periphery to centre, from *fu-past* to *now*, while the mind wanders towards the many *there-thens*, a reflection of human pathology. We live anywhere but in the *here and now*. People strive to balance this with control and perfectionism.

In sickness, sleep time flows from centre to periphery, and mind or consciousness to the here and now (logical or repetitive dreams of present issues). The resulting sleep is un-restorative.

I am confident that this lengthy article will help your sleep.

Good night!

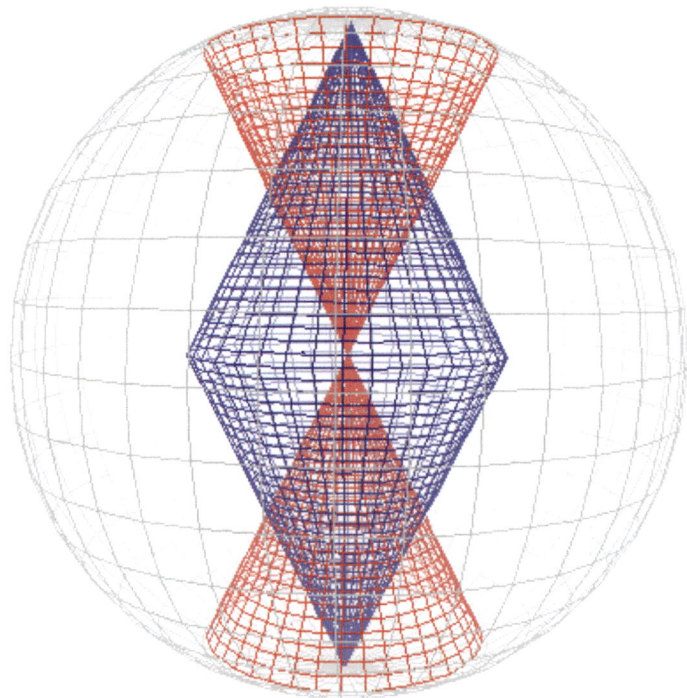

Figure 18.18 *'The Principal Symbol' the gyres, their representation as double cones with reverse flow*

References

1 Einstein A. Available online at: http://tinyurl.com/z67a4shr (accessed July 18, 2023).
2 Introduction to Masechet yevamot, Zohar. *Talmud Yerushalmi (Jerusalem Talmud)*. Available online at: http://tinyurl.com/4ys9pnn2 (accessed January 26, 2024).
3 Le Gallienne R. *Quote Investigator*. Available online at: http://tinyurl.com/2vc77fdt (accessed January 25, 2024).
4 Kiderra I. Backs to the future: Aymara language and gesture point to mirror-image view of time. *Physics*, June 12, 2006. Available online at: http://tinyurl.com/2zr9kbc8 (accessed July 17, 2023).
5 Narby J. The Cosmic Serpent: DNA and the Origins of Knowledge *Consciousness and Nature*. Available online at: http://tinyurl.com/2ds98zvu (accessed July 17, 2023e).
6 McKenna T. *The Invisible Landscape: Mind, Hallucinogen, and the I Ching*. London: Bravo Ltd, 21 June, 1994 (reprint edition).
7 The Kabbalah of Sleep. *Chabad*. Available online at: http://tinyurl.com/ffr9ss8f (accessed July 17, 2023).
8 Sherr J. *Dynamic Materia Medica of The Noble Gases: Helium*. Glasgow: Saltire Books, 2013.
9 Goertzel B. The Physics and Phenomenology of Time. *Goertzel*. Available online at: http://tinyurl.com/5n6h7964 (accessed July ????)
10 Moreva E, Brida G, Gramegna M et al. Time from quantum entanglement: An experimental illustration. *Phys. Rev. A* 89, 052122, May 2014. A. Abstract available online at: http://tinyurl.com/3ud3rcnu (accessed January 29, 2024).
11 Quantum Experiment Shows How Time Emerges from Entanglement', *New Quantum Physics*, 2013. Available online at: http://tinyurl.com/msykyt79 (accessed July 17, 2023).
12 Quantum Experiment Shows How Time Emerges from Entanglement. *Quantum Activist*. Available online at: http://tinyurl.com/msykyt79 (accessed July 17, 2023).
13 Goertzel B. On Physics and the Phenomenology of Time. *Ben Goertzel's Selected Essays and Papers*. Available online at: http://tinyurl.com/49hs7paj (accessed July 17, 2023).
14 Faccio D, Velten A, Wetzstein G. Non-line-of-sight Imaging. *Nature Reviews Physics, 318*: May 13, 2020. pp318–327. Available online at: http://tinyurl.com/yj35fc4w (accessed July 17, 2023).
15 C Everson. Sleep Deprivation in the Rat: III. Total Sleep Deprivation. *Sleep* 12(1): 1989, 13–21. Abstract available online at *Pub Med*: http://tinyurl.com/6jt9pwdm (accessed July 17, 2023).
16 Walker M. *Why we sleep: The new science of sleep and dreams*. Harlow, England: Penguin Books, 2018.
17 Wilson DR. How Long Can You Go Without Sleep? *Healthline*. Available online at: http://tinyurl.com/mweawcws (accessed July 17, 2023).

18 Eddington AS. *Wikiquote*. Available online at: http://tinyurl.com/42srz5fy (accessed July 18, 2023).

19 Second Law of Thermodynamics. *All About Science*. Available online at: http://tinyurl.com/34sxz3br (accessed July 17, 2023).

20 Buller AHR. There Was a Young Lady Named Bright Whose Speed Was Far Faster Than Light. *Quote Investigator*. Available online at: http://tinyurl.com/5566jhus (accessed July 18, 2023).

21 Cramer JG. The Quantum Handshake Explored. Available online at: http://tinyurl.com/y9d9pfpc (accessed July 17, 2023).

22 Faye J. Backward Causation. *Stanford Encyclopedia of Philosophy*. Available online at: http://tinyurl.com/4f4zy8jh (accessed July 17, 2023).

23 University of Bristol, 2021. In the Quantum Realm, Not Even Time Flows as you Might Expect. *Science Daily*. Available at: http://tinyurl.com/5fkjjmt3 (accessed July 17, 2023).

24 Loschmidt's Paradox. *Chem Europe*. Available online at: http://tinyurl.com/53d-typvv (accessed July 17, 2023).

25 Sherr J. *Sherr's Laws*. Unpublished.

26 Lao Tzu. (Trans by Gia-fu Feng and Jane English.) Chapter 48 *Tao Te Ching*. Available online at: http://tinyurl.com/593kpmkn (accessed July 18, 2023).

27 Sheldrake M. Entangled Life: How Fungi Make Our Worlds, Change Our Minds and Shape Our Futures. London: Random House, 2020.

28 Zyga L. Physicist Proposes Solution to Arrow of Time Paradox. *Phys Org*. Available online at: http://tinyurl.com/bddj4th5 (accessed July 17, 2023).

29 Carroll L. Gooreads: Lewis *Carroll Quotes*. Available online at: http://tinyurl.com/4e3j7av9 (accessed July 18, 2023).

30 Eddington A. Times Arrow, *Vinaire's Blog*, February 9, 2018. Available online at: http://tinyurl.com/yc2k9myb (accessed July 18, 2023).

31 Sherr J., *The Dynamic Materia Medica of the Noble Gases: Argon*. Glasgow: Saltire Books, 2017.

32 Hahnemann CS. *The Organon* (Sixth Edition) §15. Available online at: http://tinyurl.com/fp7ssdv6 (accessed January 30, 2024).

33 Dean J. 10 Facts About Dreaming. *Psy Blog*. Available online at: http://tinyurl.com/45k3pzys (accessed July 17, 2023).

34 Whyte C. We Dream Loads More Than We Thought. *New Scientist*, 10 April 2017. Available online at: http://tinyurl.com/5xp35hby (accessed July 17, 2023).

35 Hartle JB. The Physics of Now (February 7, 2008). *Arxiv*. Available online at: http://tinyurl.com/3bwab87s (accessed July 17, 2023).

36 *Inception* (Warner Bros, 2010). *IMDb*. Available online at: www.imdb.com/title/tt1375666/ (accessed July 18, 2023).

37 *Insomnia*. 1997. *IMDb*. Available online at: www.imdb.com/title/tt0119375/ (accessed July 18, 2023).

38 *Following*. 1998. *IMDb*. Available online at: www.imdb.com/title/tt0154506/

39 Herrick R. Dreams Poem. *PoemHunter.com*. Available online at: http://tinyurl.com/5374k5ny (accessed July 18, 2023).

40 Dreams. *Kabbalah Centre*. Available online at: http://tinyurl.com/3vmaxdzz (accessed July 18, 2023).

41 Yeats WB. The Second Coming. *Poem of the Week*. Available online at: http://tinyurl.com/yyzcwvh5 (accessed July 17, 2023).

42 Dunbar B. Scientists Report an Odd Twist near Milky Way Center, *NASA*. Available online at: http://tinyurl.com/mrz3kw8x (accessed July 17, 2023).

43 Vaze K, Sharma V. On the Adaptive Significance of Circadian Clocks for their Owners', *Research Gate*, Available online at: http://tinyurl.com/3jcx3e6y (accessed July 17, 2023).

44 Yeats WB. Geometry, *Yeat's Vision*. Available online at: http://www.yeatsvision.com/Geometry.html (accessed July 17, 2023).

45 Mann N. A Reader's Guide to Yeats: A Vision: Geometry. Available online at: http://tinyurl.com/3a6e82kt (accessed July 17, 2023).

46 Russell W. Russell Optic Dynamo-Generator. Available online at: http://tinyurl.com/28wjpd9u (accessed July 17, 2023).

47 Russell W. Generator Coils. *Rexresearch*. Available online at: http://tinyurl.com/3u885ykx (accessed July 17, 2023).

48 Mercola J. Your Body Literally Glows with Light. *Wake up World*. Available online at: http://tinyurl.com/3rj8cjsr (accessed July 17, 2023).

49 Sherr J. *The Dynamic Materia Medica of the Noble Gases: Helium*. Glasgow: Saltire Books, 2013.

50 Packard K. The Whorl – Deciphering your own Fingerprints. *American Academy of Hand Analysis*. Available online at: http://tinyurl.com/2s4hvbn7 (accessed July 17, 2023).

51 Milgrom LR. Toward a Unified Theory of Homeopathy and Conventional Medicine. *J. Alt. Comp. Med.* 13(7): Oct 2007.

52 Kent JT. Argentum Metallicum. *Lectures on Homeopathic Materia Medica*. Available online at: http://tinyurl.com/3evtrpts (accessed January 27, 2023).

19

PERIOD IV SYNTHESIS

How very noble of you

Go,
Thought Tao
First thought, limitless possibilities.
Dot banged big, shattering all eternity.
Only one miniscule fragment of singularity
Refused to scatter
Waiting for entropy to tire, retreat
Contracting universes back into one.

Tall stood the souls, poised on ledge
Spirit blew gently, and forward they leant,
Caught by carbon's gravity
They swirl the labyrinth
Of nature's destiny.
Only helium, holding his line
Refused the imperfection,
Resisted surface tension
Of
H to O, Soul binding Ego.
And so remains on high,
Manifesting nothing but
Eternal pointless sighs

Warm shone the sun,
Casting slanted shadows dawn,
Enticing
Excited buds to germinate,
Personalities to procreate.
Trees to grow high.
Neon alone, denies invagination
Clings flat earth perspective,
Cells lining the valley of despair
Baptized in superficial city lights in
Perpetual mitosis
He is born again.
And again, into tedium

Tock tick, tock tick
Time flapped its wings.
Onwards pushed the souls,
Stubbornly toiling the continuum
Argon, preserving her perfect moment
Refused to clock in
Then flawlessly decayed

Re-joice, smiled cycle
We can pause in the familiar
Recognize repetition
Recalculate direction.
But this time
Krypton
Refused to curve
Working all night
in his linear digital
Office, he rotted
in his own karma

Change, opportunity knocked,
Let's try anew,
From bird's eye view
Revisit, grow
The fruits of experience.
Xenon, at the crossroads, did not look back
Or forward. Refusing to re-evolve
His fruits shriveled bitter
Old.
X marks his grave

Jump, beckoned dot
One more step, one more battle,
Before returning home.
Radon, not daring the 7th
Rested on his laurels of power
Watched, terrified, as the
Dragon puffed fire,
Burning his castle
Into scorched ground

And luciferium?
Infinite inferno.
He collapsed in laughter.
After all, what could be funnier than hell
Or worse than his ridiculous nickname.
Oganesson? Come on!
He returned to his thankless task
Of engulfing
Countless fu-pasts
Into a singularity
To begin again.

Meanwhile
Back in the ranch
One hundred and eleven (III)
Elemental working class heroes
Break the line.
Bent, lent, spent, hunched, stooped, contorted
They struggle life's hard knock school,
Fall,
Flat on back
Reclining in submission,
Resigning disposition
They crawl the earth, barely raising weary
Bodysouls.
Some resist gravities, shake adversity, rise to challenge
And sharing their possessions
Gain height, and pride, momentum.
Only the select few
Climb the mountain peak,
Attaining with toil
That which their noble idols
inherited all too easily.
And standing tall
Align integrity
With upright pose
Non disposed
They reach up,
Flip the switch,
The universal current flows,
Connecting heaven, earth
They shine immortal.
Non inuitilis vixi
I have not lived in vain.

Some salmon never leave their mountain springs
Wallowing in comfortable convenience
They brave not river, sea, bear,
Nor leap dam
Nor swim the psoric mirror
They wait
For the sad dregs of their siblings
To return
And die.
And having never learnt a thing, they linger
Nobly frozen in spacetime's snowy mountain pools.

Period four synthesis

Feels like time is ticking away – I'm waiting for what?

Argon finally reaches maturity at 18, graduating his timeless magic garden. Captain Hook has slain Peter Pan. Krypton dives though the looking glass, clocking in at the office as a computer slave. Frontal lobes spin coded loops in a time-framed, heartless life. Dreams give way to logic, space-time bends, revolves, and repeats. Karma bites its own tail and gravity attracts alien-nation. Enter the age of chronicity.

We cannot preserve the past. The gateway to childhood's garden closes behind us, concealed by a mirror that reverses our polarities. The periodic table of our devolution is a one-way street. We are now doomed to travel down the right road in the wrong direction, driving grimly forward in reverse, hoping to arrive. The faster we go, and the harder we work, the further away we are from our destination. There is only one way to return to the source, to reverse the deadly process, and that is by finding the Tree of Life. But the Tree of Life is disguised as its mirror-image, the Tree of Knowledge, and so it cannot be found without looking through the mirror, the similimum. Paradox is a gateway to a higher truth. Meanwhile we must march the beat of time, heading down the periods towards Xenon and Beyond.

Tic tok, tok tic. Krypton bends time into the fourth dimension. Every noble gas provides an answer to a question posed by the preceding period, while at the same time posing a question to the following period. We yearn to return to the previous period, but are forced to move forward and seek new solutions.

The devolution so far can be summed up by the following sequence, a play in seven acts:

Pre-Creation singularity: I am truly One.
Hydrogen: I have lost my oneness. Alone in space.
Helium's solution: Fuse the dots into a line.
Helium' pathology: Confined to a line. Up down, up down.
Helium's question to the second period: No more up down, please.
Neon's answer: Lean forward. Divide, splitting line into width; create a two-dimensional surface.
Neon's pathology: Surface tension.
Neon's question to the third period: How can I outgrow my superficiality?
Argon's answer: Stand up tall and grow a spine, baby. Height creates space to play in.
Argon's pathology: Trying to preserve childhood's perfection, which is growing stale.
Argon's question to the fourth period: How can I move forward?
Krypton's answer: Take your time, kid.
Krypton's pathology: Time takes the kid.
Krypton' question to the fifth period: Get me off this treadmill. Unlock my clock, please.
Xenon: Jump off and restart. I know a short cut. Then you can choose.

We approach the fifth dimension. But not quite yet.

I have problems with numbers, especially 5s.
Keppler and Newton were discussing how no-one yet can draw a perfect heptagon, because it has not yet been revealed.

We will meet at the X-road.

> Time present and time past
> Are both perhaps present in time
> future,
> And time future contained in
> time past.
> TS Eliot. *The Four Quartets*[1]

The End

Reference

1   Eliot TS. Four Quartets: "Blunt Norton". *Eliot's Poetry*. Available online at: (accessed July 18, 2023).

INDEX

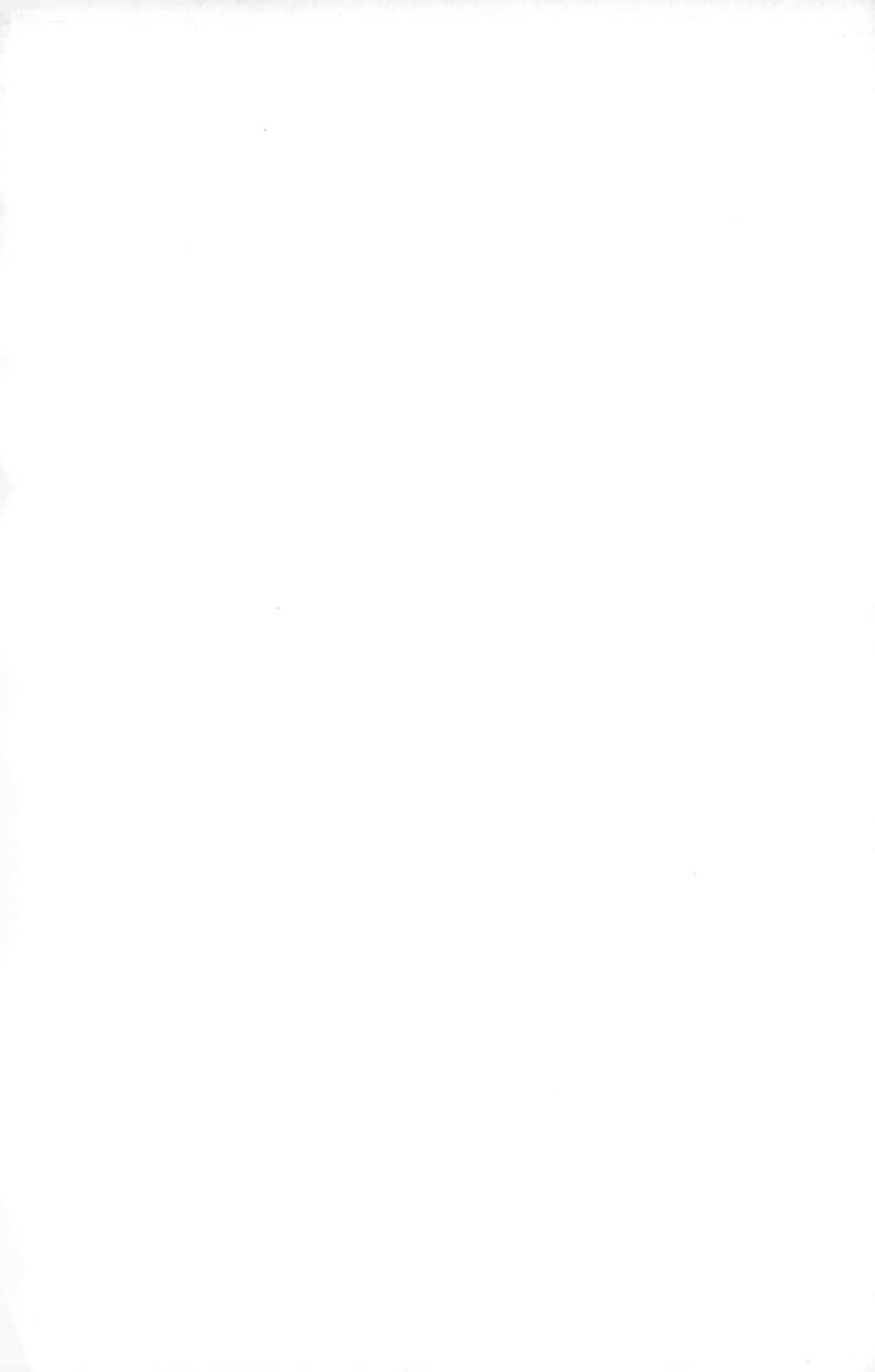